Homeopat
Medicine
for Children
and Infants

Also by Dana Ullman

Discovering Homeopathy:
Medicine for the 21st Century

Everybody's Guide to Homeopathic Medicines
(with Stephen Cummings, M.D.)

The One Minute (or so) Healer

Homeopathic Medicine for Children and Infants

~

Dana Ullman, M.P.H.

Foreword by Richard Solomon, M.D.

Jeremy P. Tarcher/Putnam
a member of
Penguin Putnam Inc.
New York

Jeremy P. Tarcher/Putnam
a member of
Penguin Putnam Inc.
375 Hudson Street
New York, NY 10014
www.penguinputnam.com

Copyright © 1992 by Dana Ullman

Published simultaneously in Canada.

Library of Congress Cataloging-in-Publication Data

Ullman, Dana.
    Homeopathic medicine for children and infants / Dana Ullman ;
  foreword by Richard Solomon.
      p.   cm.
    Includes bibliographical references (p. 251) and index.
    ISBN 0-87477-692-9
    1. Children—Diseases—Homeopathic treatment.   2. Infants—
  Diseases—homeopathic treatment.   I. Title.
  RX503.U55   1992
  615.5′32′083—dc20   92-5048
                                                           CIP

ISBN: 9780874776928

Design by Lee Fukui

Printed in the United States of America
59th Printing

~

DEDICATION

This book is dedicated to those parents who encourage their family doctor to study and use homeopathic medicines . . . if he or she doesn't do so already.

CONTENTS

~

ACKNOWLEDGMENTS

Writing this book required drawing on the wisdom and experience of two hundred years of homeopaths who built the solid foundation for this natural medicine. My thanks to every man and woman who contributed to this art and science.

Numerous homeopaths reviewed parts of this book, and I thank them for it: Randall Neustaedter, O.M.D., Michael Carlston, M.D., Ted Chapman, M.D., Jacqueline Wilson, M.D., Paul Herscu, N.D., Michael Schmidt, D.C., Louis Klein, R.S.Hom., Peggy Chipkin, F.N.P., Janet Zand, N.D., C.A., Stephen Messer, N.D., and Julian Winston; each contributed important information which was integrated into this book.

The material in this book covering the use of external homeopathic applications required detailed information about how each type of application is made. This information came from several homeopathic pharmacists including Michael Quinn, R.Ph., Mark Phillips, Sabine Hockenjos-Zogg, Forrest Murphy, and Ron Ingino.

This book also required careful reviewing of the pediatric literature. I thank pediatricians Tom Carlston, M.D., and Richard Solomon, M.D., for their important input.

A special thanks to my editor, Donna Zerner, who helped me to say what I mean and mean what I say. Not only did she edit this book with authority, she helped me to get into my readers' minds and to write with clarity and detail.

Most of all, I thank my own pediatrician, my father, Dr. Sanford Ullman. In addition to being a loving father, he encouraged the healer within me by giving me my first medical bag. Although my older brother often used one of the toy instruments to hit me with, my father taught me how to take the little white pills in the kit to help relieve the pain.

Needless to say, I have continued to use those little white pills ever since.

~

FOREWORD

More and more families are using homeopathy in America. They are discovering that this 200-year-old, internationally recognized approach to healing is safe, effective, and natural. The person most responsible for bringing homeopathy into the American spotlight is Dana Ullman, M.P.H. His first book, cowritten with Stephen Cummings, M.D., *Everybody's Guide to Homeopathic Medicines*, was a landmark publication. I recommend it (along with a first-aid kit) to my patient's parents as the indispensable first book for understanding the general approach to homeopathic treatment.

Now, I have the privilege of introducing *Homeopathic Medicine for Children and Infants* as the second indispensable book, specifically for pediatric patients. Once again, Ullman shares his remarkable ability to help families understand the inner workings of homeopathy in a simple, charming, and excellent manner.

Conventional pediatrics offers effective treatments for many serious conditions but, as every parent knows, it also has its limitations. These limitations are especially apparent in the office-based, acute care pediatric setting where greater than 90 percent of acute illnesses are viral in nature. Have you noticed your pediatrician hesitating after he or she has diagnosed a viral condition? This hesitation indicates a lack of options. Antibiotics are not effective against upper respiratory infections, influenza, or gastroenteritis. You can purchase a myriad of over-the-counter medicines, but most of them have side effects and merely suppress symptoms rather than heal your child. You could give Tylenol for your child's fever but the suppression of fever with Tylenol has been conclusively shown to hinder the immune system's response to viral infections. You could get Robitussin for your child's cough but a cough is the watchdog of the lung. Runny noses carry away millions of

xiv   HOMEOPATHIC MEDICINE FOR CHILDREN AND INFANTS

infecting viruses. Vomiting and diarrhea purge the system of disease. (Of course, the main side effect is to make drug companies rich at your child's expense.) If your pediatrician doesn't hesitate, maybe he or she should—and not just for viral infections. Homeopathy works for many other conditions as well.

Families need more options. Homeopathy is a wonderful option because homeopathic remedies are safe, cause no side effects or allergic reactions, and are inexpensive. They are easy to use because they taste good and, above all, they are curative, not suppressive. Rather than hinder the body's response to illness, homeopathy gives your child an immunological boost. This boost is just a little one. In homeopathy, extremely small amounts of natural substances are used—just enough to get your child over the hill of his or her illness. After that it's smooth sailing as your child's healing powers complete the cure. Some of the hard-headed scientists are skeptical of this microdose medicine. They say it works by placebo. But very young children don't understand the placebo effect and, as an open-minded yet skeptical pediatrician, I have seen homeopathy work decisively and consistently with infants. There is also a growing body of scientific research that confirms such clinical observations. In part 1, Ullman tells why homeopathy makes sense and describes the principles of this wonderful art and science.

If homeopathy sounds too good to be true, there is one catch—finding the right remedy. With homeopathic medicines, the keys are many and the locks are few. Like a key, the remedy must fit the lock or else you won't get in and nothing happens. But that's why this book was written—to serve as your personal guide to the discovery of the right remedy.

Unlike allopathic medicine, remedies are not based on broad categories of disease like "otitis media" or "bronchopneumonia," but on a group of symptoms. These symptoms will be unique to your child. For instance, when the flu goes through your home, each person gets the flu in his or her own way. One person has chills and is restless; another aches all over and just lies around. The key, then, in homeopathy is to find the one remedy that best fits the symptom picture. Part 2 helps you locate a set of possible remedies and then pick the right one. In part 3, the remedies are presented by the conditions they commonly cure. If your child has flu-like symptoms, for instance, you would look under "Influenza" for remedies commonly used for the flu. The symptoms of the remedy can then be matched to the symptoms of your child: Open Sesame!

In part 4, the full richness of the remedies is presented, each with their own personality, tendencies, and symptom picture. Finally, Ullman describes combination medicines for common problems and lists resources for learning more about homeopathy.

The more you learn about homeopathy, the more you will realize its depth and wisdom. While this book addresses the homeopathic approach to common, acute illnesses, it should not be used to treat chronic (constitutional) problems. For those more persistent problems, you will have to find a homeopathic practitioner who can treat your child "constitutionally."

With this brief introduction to Dana Ullman's book, I hope to have described why homeopathy is a "natural" for pediatrics. Its gentleness and effectiveness are so well suited to children that neither parents nor pediatricians should hesitate to use it.

Richard Solomon, M.D.
Assistant Professor of Pediatrics
Medical College of Pennsylvania

INTRODUCTION

Many parents consider homeopathy a godsend to their children as well as to themselves. Homeopathic medicines can be quick and effective for treating infant teething or colic, turning cranky babies into giggling cherubs. They can reduce the pain and discomfort of a child's earache, which sharply decreases the need for antibiotics or ear tubes. They can strengthen the child's own natural defenses so that he can fight off that cold or flu that every other kid in school seems to be getting. And they can benefit the hyperactive child, helping to calm his restlessness.

Homeopathic remedies are able not only to relieve many common acute problems of children but can also help to prevent recurrent bouts of illness. And homeopathic medicines can treat both physical ailments and emotional upsets.

With the aid of this book, all of these valuable benefits are within your grasp.

OUR CHILDREN/OURSELVES

A growing number of parents are concerned about the side effects of conventional drugs, especially in the treatment of babies and young children. Lynn and Ken Elliot of Berkeley, California, are two such parents. While they seek out their pediatrician for their baby Elizabeth's general check-ups and for diagnosis of potentially dangerous symptoms, they also feel that the best medical care often begins in the home. Instead of rushing Elizabeth to the pediatrician every time she coughs, or has a cold, fever, or earache, Lynn and Ken use homeopathic medicines to treat her themselves.

Although both are relatively new to homeopathy, they

have used these natural medicines successfully for treating many common pediatric complaints. They first tried homeopathy when Elizabeth was four months old. She had colic and was crying intensely. Although Elizabeth's discomfort was relieved when she was carried and rocked, she would immediately begin wailing as soon as she was put back in her crib. After a couple of hours, even the carrying and rocking didn't help, and Elizabeth cried almost constantly.

Ken and Lynn then remembered that a friend had given them a book on homeopathy at Elizabeth's baby shower and, after reviewing the chapter on colic, they got *Chamomilla 30* (chamomile) from their homeopathic medicine kit, crushed a couple of small pellets between two spoons to make them easy for Elizabeth to swallow, and put them under her tongue. Within a minute or so Elizabeth was asleep and, upon waking, her colic was gone.

Although this may sound like a miracle cure, such miracles are common when using homeopathic medicines. Of course, such dramatic successes don't happen every time: homeopathy, like every kind of healing, has its limitations. Still, its effectiveness as well as its safety are recognized today by millions of people all over the world.

In fact, homeopathic medicine, for many reasons, has achieved such popularity in Europe that it is no longer considered an alternative medicine there. First, England's Royal Family has been under homeopathic care since the 1830s. Second, organized medicine in Europe has not been as antagonistic to homeopathy as American medical organizations have been. And third, convincing research has been published in numerous European medical and scientific journals.

One-third of the French population uses homeopathic medicines, and 32 percent of French family physicians prescribe them. One-fifth of all German physicians use homeopathic medicines; 42 percent of British physicians refer patients to homeopathic physicians, and 45 percent of Dutch physicians consider homeopathic medicines effective. If these figures aren't impressive enough, according to a recent market research survey by London's Frost and Sullivan Ltd., the field of alternative and complementary medicine, including homeopathy, is expanding so quickly that it was Europe's second biggest growth industry during the 1980s, second only to the computer industry. ("Complementary medicine" is a term popularized by Prince Charles to emphasize that much of alternative medicine is not simply an alternative but is a valid complement to other types of medical care.)

Many people in England who grew up with homeopathy are now having their own children who they regularly treat homeopathically. Such is the case with Terry and Diane Linden, who live in London and whose three children (five, eleven, and fifteen years of age) have been brought up using homeopathic medicines. Two of these children have never taken a conventional drug, and the other child has done so on only a couple of occasions.

Terry and Diane have noticed that many of their friends' children—treated with conventional medicines—would get recurrent bouts of their symptoms. The antibiotics that were used to treat sore throats or ear infections would have to be used again and again. Terry and Diane questioned if conventional drugs were really curative or simply acting on the symptoms alone.

Terry and Diane's children get sick occasionally just like other children, but with the aid of homeopathic medicines, they get over their illnesses relatively quickly and don't generally have recurrent bouts of the same illnesses. What's more, Terry and Diane have begun to teach their two older children how to use homeopathic medicines themselves to treat common ailments and injuries. By teaching their children how to care for themselves with homeopathic medicines, these parents are empowering their children in a way that is in itself therapeutic.

Using safer, natural remedies, such as homeopathic medicines, is particularly important when treating infants and young children. Their young bodies are developing. Their nervous systems are just beginning to integrate with the endocrine and immune systems and with various organ systems. Although the human organism can be incredibly resilient, it can also be very fragile, especially during infancy.

Parents can be reassured that homeopathic medicines are safe for infants. Despite the fact that some homeopathic remedies are made from originally poisonous substances, they are diluted so many times that it is not possible for a baby to ingest enough of the substance to cause any damage, even if the infant swallowed the contents of an entire bottle.

To make it easier for infants to take a dose of a homeopathic medicine, you should crush the pellets or pills between two clean spoons and then place the powder in the baby's mouth. Because homeopathic medicines are made with a small amount of lactose (milk sugar) or sucrose, they have a sweet taste that most infants and children love. (Although some parents may be trying to restrict the amount of lactose and sucrose in their children's diet, the amount contained in homeopathic medicines is so small that it poses no real problem, even for diabetic children.)

~

THE NEED FOR SAFE ALTERNATIVES

Parents tend to be more concerned about their children's diet, safety, and hygiene than they are about their own, and are inclined to seek out quality health care for their children, even for minor complaints. Unfortunately, parental concern too often translates into anxiety and fear, preventing parents from taking constructive action at home. Instead, many parents with a sick child immediately take their child to a doctor, even for minor ailments, hoping that the doctor will simply make the problem go away.

The care that conventional physicians offer is often valuable, but powerful drugs are dispensed far too frequently by too many doctors without an effort to try safer, more natural

xx   HOMEOPATHIC MEDICINE FOR CHILDREN AND INFANTS

therapies. It seems prudent to save the bigger guns for the more serious conditions that warrant their use.

Dr. Joe Graedon, pharmacologist and author of *The People's Pharmacy*, warns parents and doctors about prescribing drugs to infants and children: "Their immature organ systems often deal with drugs much differently than their grown-up version will a few years later, and the differences can lead to anything from uncomfortable reactions to deadly ones."

The short-term effects of most drugs on infants and children are often unknown, and the long-term effects are not simply unknown but can be frightening. A 1990 study by the United States Government's General Accounting Office reviewed the 198 new drugs which were approved by the Food and Drug Administration between 1976 and 1985. The study discovered that more than half of these drugs caused serious reactions that had gone undetected until several years after widespread use. The report also showed that the drugs reviewed by the FDA for use by children were twice as likely to lead to serious reactions as those approved for use by adults. Some of the most severe reactions included heart failure, anaphylactic shock, convulsions, kidney and liver failure, severe blood disorders, birth defects, blindness, and even death. The seriousness of these side effects is enough to send chills up any parent's spine; hopefully, parents and physicians will soon understand the importance of using conventional drugs more conservatively.

Most people do not realize that many conventional drugs are not tested on children. The safety and effectiveness of giving drugs to children have not been established. When it comes to calculating doses or anticipating side effects, children are not little adults.

Additional risks arise when a physician prescribes more than one drug at a time. Surveys have shown that over 20 percent of all visits to a doctor by children under fifteen years of age include a prescription for two or more drugs per visit. Many types of drugs, which may be relatively safe when given alone, can become dangerous when prescribed along with another drug. The long-term effect of giving certain drugs to infants, especially two or more drugs at a time, remains unknown.

This kind of overprescribing is sometimes the result of inadequate knowledge of recent research. It also sometimes occurs because a doctor feels compelled to prescribe something for a sick child. Doctors often assume that the medicine, even if not certain to be effective, will at least have a beneficial placebo effect. However, considering the potential side effects from nearly every drug, it seems more prudent to consider more mild placebos or safer medicines, such as homeopathic remedies.

Children often resist taking a conventional medicine. Perhaps they are trying to tell us something. Perhaps they know something that their physician and their parents don't. (It is interesting to note that veterinarians who practice homeopathic medicine have commonly observed that animals seem to be less frightened when they are treated with homeopathic remedies than when they are given conventional drugs.)

Whether children actually know or sense that homeopathic medicines are good for them or not, they deserve safe medicines. It is time that parents and physicians seek safe, natural, and effective alternatives to conventional, potentially harmful drugs. Homeopathic medicine is one such alternative.

HOW TO USE THIS BOOK

The first part of this book will give you an overview of homeopathy: what it is, how it works, the similarities and differences between homeopathy and conventional medicine, as well as homeopathy's limitations. The second part will teach you basic principles of homeopathy and how to use the medicines with the greatest effectiveness. It will teach you the important questions you need to ask in order to find the correct remedy, how to determine the best potency and dosage, what to avoid while taking a homeopathic medicine, and how to store your homeopathic medicines.

Part 3, "Common Ailments of Children," will probably be the section of the book you refer to the most. This is an alphabetized listing of common ailments and injuries and it describes the homeopathic medicines most frequently used in treating them. To find the best remedy for your child's ailment, you will look for the description of the homeopathic medicine that most closely fits the unique pattern of your child's symptoms.

Part 4, "Essential Homeopathic Medicines," provides information about the most commonly used homeopathic medicines, their unique typologies, origins, and the physical and psychological symptoms for which each is prescribed. This will help you to choose a medicine more accurately. If you are having trouble pinpointing the correct remedy after you have looked up the specific ailment in part 3, pick out the top two to four medicines that best describe your child's symptoms, and then read about each of these medicines in further depth in part 4. (Not every medicine listed in part 3 will be in part 4, since only the most commonly used remedies have been described. For more information about remedies not listed in this section, see one of the books with what is called a *materia medica*, listed in the Resources section.)

Part 5, "Commercial Homeopathic Medicines," describes many of the common homeopathic medicines that are found in health food stores and pharmacies. It will give you an overview of the many combination medicines that are readily available on today's market, and the advantages and disadvantages of using these products are discussed.

Part 5 also includes a section on external homeopathic applications. Most homeopathic medicines are used for internal consumption because healing is best stimulated from the inside. There are, however, numerous types of external homeopathic applications used for cuts, abrasions, burns, bites, sprains, and strains. Each type of external application, whether it is a tincture, ointment, gel, cream, or lotion, has certain advantages and disadvantages. This section will help you determine what type of external application is best for your child's particular injury.

The Appendix includes a short review of research on homeopathy, which may not only be of interest to those who use homeopathic medicines but to the various friends, family members, and medical personnel who may be skeptical about this different form of medicine.

The Appendix also includes a list of each homeopathic medicine referred to in this book along with a guide to its pronunciation. Homeopathic medicines are known by their Latin names, which are sometimes difficult to pronounce; this guide may help.

I hope this book stimulates you to learn more about homeopathy and encourages you to use homeopathic medicines at home. The Resources section will help you explore further. It gives you a source list of the best homeopathic books, manufacturers, organizations, and training programs.

PROFESSIONAL HOMEOPATHIC CARE

The medicines described in this book are primarily useful for the acute or short-term phase of most illnesses. For instance, you will often be able to help relieve your child's sore throat, cold, allergy, headache, or insomnia. However, if your child has recurrent bouts of these conditions, I strongly recommend you seek professional homeopathic care, which may be able to cure the chronic ailment that underlies the symptoms.

Treating the underlying disease often requires what is called *constitutional homeopathic care*. After careful analysis of the child's heredity, health history, and complete physical, emotional, and mental symptoms, the professional homeopath prescribes an individualized homeopathic medicine that is often able to promote a deep cure of a chronic disease. Although constitutional care will not *always* cure a chronic ailment, it is often successful in at least reducing the severity and intensity of your child's complaints.

This book will not teach you how to treat every illness that your infant or child will have; there are serious health problems that clearly require the care of a physician. And, while many of these more serious conditions—such as pneumonia, epilepsy, and diabetes—can be positively affected by homeopathic medicines, their treatment requires significantly more information about homeopathy and pathology than is offered in this book. Seek the care of a professionally trained homeopath for such conditions (see the Resources section).

This book does not provide much information on how to treat many common skin conditions of children. Homeopaths believe that skin symptoms are the result of internal problems which often require constitutional care. There are so many homeopathic medicines that can be potentially useful for these conditions that it is difficult for untrained people to accurately determine the correct medicine. The skin conditions that *are* covered in this book are diaper rash, impetigo, and herpes. The reason these exceptions are made is because each of these conditions has a certain limited number of homeopathic medicines that are commonly effective in treating them. Still, although it may be relatively easy to heal the acute symptoms of these skin conditions, a permanent cure may require constitutional care.

Despite the great power of homeopathic medicines, their use does not replace basic principles of healthy living: diet, exercise, hygiene, environment, and psychological factors all affect a child's health. Proper care and attention to these influences can both prevent and heal disease. Homeopathic medicine should simply complement healthy living. Although homeopathy is not the only means of children's health care, it is an important and sometimes vital art and science of healing.

Homeopathic
Medicine
for Children
and Infants

PART 1

Why Homeopathy Makes Sense

THE WISDOM OF THE BODY

The human body performs miracles every day, every hour, every second. To survive, it must continually defend itself against bacteria, viruses, poisons, allergens, environmental stresses, psychological stresses, and the innumerable seen and unseen influences that attack it.

The body has developed sophisticated means of responding to these assaults. It creates fever and inflammation to burn out invading germs and isolate foreign substances. It develops nasal discharge to help excrete dead viruses and dead white blood cells. It uses pain to draw attention to an injured or diseased part that needs to be rested or treated.

The body creates symptoms as its way to both adapt to stress or infection as well as to defend and ultimately heal itself. This response is not conscious. We do not have to tell the body to heal itself. It is an automatic response, an inherent wisdom; the body seems to know precisely how to fight disease and heal injuries, and it has done this millions of times before. It has survived up to now due to this impressive ability to defend itself and to adapt to its changing environment. Still, each body has its limitations.

Despite the glorious perfection of the human form, it, like any living organism, is prone to illness. It will not win every battle against infection. It will not successfully adapt to every environmental insult. It will not effectively withstand every new stress.

Still, a person's symptoms represent his body's best efforts to defend and heal itself. Because of this, it does not make sense to inhibit these natural defenses. Treatments that suppress symptoms may be temporarily successful but will inevitably be ineffective in promoting health; such treatments are not physiologically sound.

The body tells us that suppressing symptoms doesn't really cure a person. Not only may symptoms return, they often return with more vehemence; or maybe worse, they don't return, but other more serious symptoms take their place. Recognizing the wisdom of the body is vital for anyone interested in healing. Ignoring this wisdom too often results in using treatments that are either not effective, are only temporarily effective, or have more serious side effects than they have healing benefits.

~

UNDERSTANDING SIDE EFFECTS

From a purely pharmacological point of view, there are no such things as side effects. Drugs simply have effects, and we arbitrarily differentiate those effects that we like from those that we don't like, calling the ones we don't like *side effects*.

Consider, for a moment, the conventional treament when a child has a cold. A child's body, like that of an adult, responds to cold viruses by creating increased numbers of white blood cells that fight the viruses. Some white blood cells and viruses die in this battle, so the body creates mucus as a liquid vehicle to discharge this dead matter.

Over-the-counter cold medications work either by blocking mucus formation and drying mucous membranes or by shrinking swollen nasal capillaries. Once mucus formation is blocked, the child is less able to discharge the dead viruses and white blood cells. The discharge becomes less watery and more sticky, making it difficult to blow out of the nose or cough up. It is predictable that this suppression usually results in even more disturbing symptoms. Instead of having nasal discharge, the child will often experience a congestive headache as well as various other side effects, including mental dullness, drowsiness, and in some cases hallucinations, fears, and behavioral problems.

These symptoms are not *side* effects but are the direct effects of a drug working against the body's natural healing response.

The decongestant cold medicines, which act by shrinking swollen nasal capillaries, work, but only temporarily. Although they may effectively eliminate the nasal discharge and clear the breathing passageways, once the medication is stopped all the symptoms quickly return, usually worse than before. Parents are often afraid to stop giving these drugs to the child for fear of having the symptoms return. Over time, however, the dose previously used to treat symptoms becomes less effective, and stronger doses are needed.

The worsening of symptoms after the medication is stopped—called the rebound effect—is not a side effect. It is the body trying to heal itself, which it will do more effectively if and when we stop trying to suppress its natural efforts.

Since symptoms are an important defense of the body, it makes sense to use methods that support this defense rather than those that inhibit it. Homeopathy is one such method.

UNDERSTANDING HOMEOPATHY

Homeopathic medicine is a natural pharmaceutical science that uses very small doses of substances from the plant, mineral, and animal kingdom to stimulate the body's own defenses. The homeopathic treatment for the common cold provides a simple example. One of the common homeopathic remedies for a cold is *Allium cepa,* made from the common onion. Because onions make our noses run and our eyes tear, they can aid the body in flushing out the cold virus by further stimulating processes the body is already using. As opposed to drugs that dry up mucous membranes and temporarily suppress the natural healing abilities of the body, *Allium cepa,* or any other correctly chosen homeopathic medicine, helps the body in its effort to heal itself by supporting what the body is already doing.

Allium cepa is not the only homeopathic medicine effective in treating the common cold. An important part of homeopathy is individualization. No single medicine is prescribed for everybody's cold or illness. Because the symptoms of one child's illness are likely to be different than another's, the choice of a homeopathic medicine is based upon each unique pattern of symptoms rather than on the illness itself. This individualization of symptoms is one of the important principles of homeopathy. Homeopaths individualize a medicine to a sick person based on *the law of similars.*

Principle 1: The Law of Similars

The word *homeopathy* is derived from two Greek words: *homoios* which means "similar" and *pathos* which means "disease" or "suffering." The primary principle of homeopathy is the law of similars, that is, the principle that a substance will help to heal symptoms similar to those it is known to cause. Literally any substance, plant, mineral, or animal can become a homeopathic medicine. Experiments called *provings* are done with the substance on healthy people to determine what pattern of symptoms it causes, when given in a dose sufficient to cause those symptoms. (Sick people are not used in provings because it is difficult to differentiate the symptoms of the illness from those of the substance being tested.)

It may be startling to learn that many of the most common homeopathic medicines are made from poisons. Arsenic, poison ivy, and bee venom are but a few of the remedies frequently used in homeopathic medicine. But because homeo-pathic manufacturers use these substances only in extremely small doses, they are widely recognized as safe. The FDA des-ignates homeopathic medicines over-the-counter drugs— available to anyone without a prescription—and throughout the world other countries similarly recognize the safety of ho-meopathic medicines.

Arsenic is a poison which causes a type of diarrhea that resembles food poisoning; food poisoning is but one of the conditions for which it is given in homeopathic dosage (*Arsen-icum album*). Poison ivy (*Rhus tox*), in homeopathic doses, is a remedy for certain skin rashes, since it causes them. It's also effective for sprains and strains; homeopathic provings have shown that poison ivy, taken internally, creates pains in mus-cles, tendons, and ligaments that are similar to that of a sprain.

Bee venom (*Apis mellifica*) is used homeopathically for in-flammatory conditions which are typified by burning and stinging pain. Still, like all homeopathic remedies, it must be suited to the individual. Just as it is helpful to apply ice to a bee sting, those who will benefit from homeopathic doses of bee venom are those who feel better putting ice on their inflamma-tion and are aggravated by heat. *Apis* is a common medicine for children with tonsillitis, but only when the child feels bet-ter sucking on an ice cube or prefers drinking cold drinks.

The same year that homeopathy's founder, Dr. Samuel Hahnemann, first wrote about this science, Dr. Edward Jenner first proposed using a cowpox vaccine to immunize against smallpox. The premise of immunization resembles the basic homeopathic principle of the law of similars: use small doses of a substance that causes a disease in order to stimulate the body's immune system to build a natural resistance to the disease.

Although immunizations are only used as a means of pre-vention, conventional medicine also sometimes uses the law of similars in a treatment; allergy treatment, for example. Al-lergists give patients small doses of a substance that triggers an allergic response in order to build better resistance to that substance. Another example is ritalin, being prescribed by some doctors to calm hyperactive children. Ritalin is an amphetamine-like drug that may cause hyperactivity when given to nonhyperactive children.

Although immunizations, allergy treatments, ritalin, and some other conventional drugs may be based on the law of similars, these are not considered homeopathic drugs; they are not prescribed with the same precision of individuality, nor are they prescribed in the safer, extremely small doses common to homeopathic medicines. Still, it is encouraging to see the application of at least some homeopathic principles in mainstream medicine.

Principle 2: Recognizing the Pattern of Symptoms

The concept of a *pattern of symptoms* is important in homeopathy. A person's disease is not simply one isolated symptom, but is the combination of all the physical, emotional, and mental symptoms that person is experiencing.

Homeopaths have found that every plant, mineral, or animal substance causes, in overdose, its own unique pattern of symptoms in the human body. Although there are numerous substances that cause headaches, some cause them in the back part of the head, some over the forehead, and others on one side or the other. Some substances cause headaches that are relieved by hot applications, others by cold applications; some cause pain when a person moves, others when lying flat; some create concurrent irritability, others concurrent depression. And on and on.

Just as no substance causes simply one symptom, no disease simply has one symptom. Each illness has a pattern of symptoms. One child may have a headache that is worse in the morning; another's may be worse late at night. The first child may experience relief from pressure applied to the head; the other will be aggravated by it. One child may feel restless during the headache; the other may feel lethargic.

Homeopathy recognizes that certain bodymind patterns of symptoms are common. These patterns include aspects of personality, body type, acute and chronic physical symptoms, and genetic inheritance.

Homeopaths refer to "*Sulphur* types," "*Phosphorus* types," or "*Pulsatilla* types." Each type refers to the pattern of physical, emotional, and mental symptoms that a person has had for several years—or even decades. The remedy that fits a person's type is called a *constitutional remedy*. Part 4 of this book provides basic information on some of the most common constitutional types of children. (A more detailed discussion of eight of the most common children's types is available in Paul Herscu's *The Homeopathic Treatment of Children: Pediatric Constitutional Types.*)

Knowing a child's constitutional remedy is of great value; it can be used to treat both acute and chronic ailments, and it can prevent future problems. It's also useful because it helps you better understand your child. By learning about certain traits of your child's type, you may also discover some previously unrecognized tendencies of your child.

This book, however, does not focus on teaching you to find the constitutional remedy for your child; such an effort requires more training in the system of homeopathy than a single book can offer. Instead, it teaches you how to find the correct homeopathic medicine to match the pattern of symptoms of the acutely sick child.

Principle 3:
The Use of Very Small Doses of Medicines

One of the reasons homeopathic medicines are considered safe is because such small doses of a substance are used. The medicines are made by a specific pharmacological process called *potentization*. A substance from the plant, mineral, or animal kingdom is diluted in distilled water—usually one part of the substance to nine parts water—and then the entire solution is vigorously shaken.

This process is repeated several times, each time further diluting the original mixture. When the process is completed three times, the solution is labeled 3x; when it is completed twelve times, it is called 12x, and so on.

When a substance is diluted one part to ninety-nine parts distilled water and the process is repeated three times, it is called 3c; when it is repeated twelve times, it is called 12c, and so on.

According to present laws of physics, once a substance is diluted to 24x or 12c, there should in all probability be no more molecules left of the original substance. And yet, homeopaths and homeopathic patients have observed for the past two hundred years that the more a substance is potentized—that is, the more it is diluted—the stronger and longer it acts *and* the fewer doses are needed.

It is this principle of extremely small doses that generates the greatest controversy surrounding homeopathy. Skeptics attack this concept, saying that such small doses could not possibly have any effect; homeopathic medicines are simply placeboes. Most of these skeptics, however, have never used homeopathic medicines, and most are so unfamiliar with homeopathy they cannot even describe its basic principles. Such attacks are anything but scientific.

Admittedly, it is difficult to understand how such small doses could have such powerful effects, and yet, a growing amount of research (see "Homeopathic Research" in the Appendix) and an immense amount of clinical and personal experience have verified their effectiveness.

There are numerous examples from nature which can help us to understand this phenomena. Sharks, for instance, can sense tiny amounts of blood in the water from a great distance. Male insects will travel long distances to find a female. Numerous animals emit pheromones—sexual hormones that attract the opposite sex—and again, sometimes over great distance. It is commonly recognized that insects and animals need to smell only a very small number of molecules of a substance in order to recognize it.

Ironically, although virtually every animal on the planet has incredible senses, skeptics of homeopathy assume that human beings can only sense or be affected by what can be actually seen or measured.

Still, small doses of a substance will not have any effect on an organism unless that organism is hypersensitive to it; the way to discover this hypersensitivity is through the law of similars. For instance, an insect will only be attracted to pheromones of an insect of its own species. A sick child will be sensitive to a microdose of a specific medicine only if that medicine causes a corresponding set of symptoms when given to a healthy person.

How the extremely small doses used in homeopathy actually work remains a mystery; yet, why certain conventional drugs work also remains a mystery. Only recently have scientists begun to better understand how and why aspirin works—thanks to millions of dollars of research. This ignorance did not deter physicians or patients from using aspirin; most people simply want to use whatever is effective, whether or not they understand how or why it works.

Principle 4: Understanding the Healing Process

Homeopaths are in a unique position to understand the process of healing because they interview each patient in extreme detail. They do not simply diagnose a child's specific disease but examine in detail the unique pattern of physical and psychological symptoms the child has.

Homeopaths ask how each symptom is affected by temperature, weather, time of day, motion, position, external stimuli, eating or drinking, sleep, urination or defecation, emotional or mental states, and other factors. They ask a wide range of questions to uncover the individual way that each child experiences his illness.

With the careful observation of both obvious and subtle symptoms the homeopath is better able to understand the evolution of a child's health. Also, because most homeopaths are family physicians, they are familiar with and can better treat conditions that run in the family.

As a holistic system homeopathy recognizes the physical, emotional, and mental levels of a person. Each level has a different intensity of symptoms, and each level can restrict or augment a person's experience of health.

On the physical level, diseases of the brain, nervous system, and heart represent the most serious physical problems, while conditions of the skin, muscles, and connective tissue represent the least serious physical conditions.

On the emotional level, fear of death, suicidal depression, and powerful rage represent deep emotional distress, while mild irritability, slight frustration, and simple anxiety represent the least disturbing emotional states.

On a mental level, confusion, delusional states, and identity crises represent deep stresses, while slight memory loss, temporary concentration problems, and occasional absent-mindedness represent the least disruptive mental states.

Homeopaths consider mental symptoms to be the deepest, those at the core of the person—though a symptom on *any* level can be considered deep if it is intense enough. Although some pop psychologists believe that a person's emotions represent their core being, homeopaths believe that the mental level—which consists of a person's will, understanding, and a sense of self—is the deepest part of the human being.

Recognizing these different levels becomes important in understanding the healing process. After taking a homeopathic medicine, some people experience a *healing crisis:* a situation in which certain symptoms get worse while others are relieved. Symptoms that affect the vital organs may be relieved, while more superficial symptoms are heightened. For instance, a child with a high fever and digestive symptoms may exerience an increase in diarrhea, while the potentially more serious symptom of high fever decreases. Although the diarrhea may be discomforting, it is actually demonstrating the body's efforts to heal itself.

Children and adults more often experience a healing crisis

during chronic ailments rather than during acute conditions. Recognizing that a healing crisis sometimes may occur may help relieve some parental anxiety when certain symptoms improve while others worsen. Most often, however, parents who prescribe homeopathic medicine for their children's acute ailments will simply see the medicines speed up the healing process.

Over the past two hundred years homeopaths have observed that healing progresses through three parameters, called *Hering's Law of Cure*. (Hering's Law of Cure is named after Constantine Hering, M.D., the father of American homeopathy, who was the first to describe these three parameters.)

1) *Healing first benefits internal, vital function and then progresses to external, superficial functions.* Symptoms affecting the organism's most vital functions, such as the brain and heart, usually improve first in the process of healing, while symptoms affecting the less vital functions of the body are usually the last to be relieved. In fact, the symptoms affecting the body's less vital functions may temporarily worsen in the process of cure. For instance, a child with asthma may temporarily experience a skin rash after getting relief from the asthma itself. Likewise, a child with a dry cough may, as he continues to heal, begin to cough up mucus. This coughing may alarm parents, but the now productive nature of the cough is actually helping to eliminate the mucus, ultimately clearing the child's respiratory tract. If a child has mental and emotional problems along with certain physical symptoms, the child will *generally* feel relief of the psychological symptoms prior to improvement in the physical symptoms, unless the physical symptoms are of a serious nature.

2) *Healing progresses in reverse order of its appearance.* A child with a chronic disease who is given the correct homeopathic remedy may show symptoms that she had in an earlier stage of the illness. Sometimes these symptoms may be the first symptoms she had. Sometimes these symptoms have been suppressed by conventional medical treatments. Other times the symptoms were there in infancy. This retracing of symptoms is a good sign, indicating that a deep curative process is occurring. (This is more commonly seen in the treatment of chronic disease; it is rarely experienced in children with an acute illness.)

3) *Healing progresses from the upper part of the body to the lower part.* A child with a skin rash, for example, will show relief in the upper part of the body first and then the lower part.

When this direction in healing is not followed, it is commonly assumed that the child is reacting to a placebo, experiencing only a temporary relief of symptoms, rather than a truly curative process.

Hering's Law of Cure confirms generally accepted principles of natural healing. In true healing, symptoms do not always disappear simultaneously; there is a certain order and process to the healing. Chinese medicine and naturopathic medicine have long recognized principles similar to those established in Hering's Law.

LIMITATIONS AND RISKS OF HOMEOPATHY

Homeopathic medicines cannot do everything. They cannot help a child grow back a lost limb. They cannot help a child regenerate brain cells which have been damaged or lost due to illness. And they cannot repair certain conditions such as a hernia or a ruptured appendix for which surgery may be the only appropriate treatment.

For some ailments, benefits from homeopathic medicine can only occur if other proper medical care is also provided. For instance, homeopathic medicines can help mend a fracture faster as long as the bones have been correctly set. If a child is having abdominal problems as the result of a twisted colon, a homeopathic medicine can only help once the child's problem is surgically corrected.

Also, because it is sometimes hard to find the individualized homeopathic medicine for every sick child, it can occasionally be difficult to provide a cure, even for some common, nonlife-threatening chronic diseases or acute illnesses. Children who are taking strong medications are often more difficult to treat because their natural symptoms are masked by the drugs. And since infants cannot always clearly communicate their symptoms, finding the correct remedy for them can also sometimes be difficult.

Homeopathic medicines can be effective in treating various infections in infants and children. However, if a child has a particularly high fever or some other life-threatening condition, a homeopath may want to prescribe an antibiotic or other conventional drug concurrent with a homeopathic remedy, or refer the patient to a physician who can. Recommending conventional drugs to treat infections does not suggest that homeopathic medicines are ineffective in treating these conditions, but that sometimes it is safest to combine conventional and homeopathic treatments. Some experienced homeopaths, however, will prescribe only a homeopathic medicine, and only if it does not act very rapidly will they resort to conventional therapies.

Sometimes it takes time to find the correct, individually chosen homeopathic remedy. Certain urgent pediatric conditions demand immediate treatment. In such instances, it may be prudent to give a conventional drug immediately and then later give the indicated homeopathic remedy.

Homeopathy can also be inappropriate when there is some obvious factor causing the problem. If, for instance, a child is anemic because he is severely malnourished, a homeopathic remedy will be of little value. If a child is being exposed to a poisonous substance in the home or environment, a homeopathic medicine may help the child more effectively excrete this poison but ultimately will be ineffective if the child is repeatedly exposed to this substance.

The greatest risk from using homeopathic medicines is that a parent using them may delay getting professional medical help at the times when it is warranted. To avoid such a situation, it is highly recommended to have a family health guidebook on hand, such as *Care for Your Baby and Your Child*, edited by Steven Shelov, or *Dr. Spock's Baby and Child Care*, by Benjamin Spock and Michael Rothenberg. These books provide guidelines for determining when professional medical care is essential or recommended.

A small risk from homeopathic medicines arises when parents continue to give a homeopathic remedy to their child after it has proven helpful and the symptoms have disappeared. Parents then risk having their child experience a proving of the medicine, that is, the temporary creation of symptoms when a substance is taken in sufficient amounts. Such symptoms are rarely serious and tend to disappear shortly after the medicine is stopped.

Homeopathic medicines have limitations just like any other therapy. Still, as famed violinist and philanthropist Yehudi Menuhin once said, "Homeopathy is one of the few medical specialties which carries no penalties—only benefits."

It is no wonder that five-year-old Erin Thomas said to her mother, "I like that ho-ho-ho medicine. Did Santa Claus invent it?"

Homeopathy is indeed a gift. Use it and give it to others, and we will all be healthier for it.

PART 2

How to Use Homeopathic Medicines

~

It is more important to know what kind of person has a disease than what kind of disease a person has.

Sir William Osler

Homeopathic medicines are a safe and powerful method of healing ailments and injuries. The challenge is to find the correct remedy.

This book will help you find the correct individualized homeopathic medicine for your child quickly and easily. Look up your child's ailment in part 3, "Common Ailments of Children." Read about each medicine described under the ailment; then determine which one best describes the symptoms your child is experiencing. (For more detailed information about the most commonly used remedies, see part 4.)

However, make certain you first read this part, part 2, carefully; before you can choose the correct remedy, you must first understand how to individualize the medicine for your child. This part will teach you what questions to ask your child (or what questions you need to answer for your infant) to get the information you need to find the correct homeopathic remedy. It will also teach you which symptoms are more important than others and how to choose the appropriate dose and potency of a homeopathic medicine.

Although this book will teach you which homeopathic medicine to give for most common acute childhood ailments,

15

there are additional homeopathic resources which can improve the accuracy of your remedy selection and expand the number and the kind of conditions you can successfully treat: a *repertory* and a *materia medica.* A repertory is a listing of almost every symptom you can imagine, and next to each symptom is a list of homeopathic medicines that are known to cure it. *Materia medica* is Latin for "materials of medicine"; this is a listing of medicines with descriptions of which symptoms they are known to effectively treat. (Part 4 of this book is a short *materia medica;* other more technical homeopathic books provide more detailed information.)

By using a repertory, you reduce the possible choices for the correct remedy down to a handful. Then, by reading about each of the possible remedies in a *materia medica* or in this book, you will be able to find the one individual remedy that most closely fits your child's pattern of symptoms.

The best single book that contains both a repertory and a *materia medica* is Dr. William Boericke's *Pocket Manual of Materia Medica with Repertory.*

ASSESSING THE CHILD'S
UNIQUE SYMPTOMS

Homeopaths try to discover the idiosyncratic symptoms of the ailing person, asking detailed questions in order to find the remedy that best fits the ailment. As a part of this case-taking process, homeopaths define the word *symptom* very broadly. A symptom can be:

• any pain or discomfort

• any change from what that person normally experiences

• any limitation on what that person can normally do

• anything that makes a pain or discomfort better or worse

It is not always enough to simply match one of your child's symptoms with one symptom that a medicine is known to cure. Generally, a medicine is more likely to be effective if it matches the complete pattern of symptoms the child is experiencing. It is not necessary to find a medicine that fits every symptom, but it should match the most important symptoms.

Homeopaths define four types of symptoms:

1. *Common Symptoms.* Common symptoms are those symptoms which fit a specific conventional medical diagnosis. Fever with influenza, jaundice with hepatitis, and wheezing with asthma are all common symptoms related to a specific disease. These symptoms are of *least* importance in selecting a homeopathic medicine.

2. *Local Symptoms.* A local symptom is pain or discomfort specific to a specific part of the body. A headache, a sore throat, and a cough are simple examples. Local symptoms may also be cold toes, a sweaty head, or tired eyes. Although local symptoms are important when selecting a remedy, they are not considered to be as important as general symptoms.

3. *General Symptoms.* General symptoms are those which affect the entire body. When a child is hungry or thirsty, restless or easily startled, or experiences emotional or mental distress, these are considered general symptoms because the pain or discomfort are not localized to a specific part of the body. Sleep disorders, level of energy, and sensitivity to temperature and weather are other examples of general symptoms. General symptoms

are of greater importance than local symptoms because they represent the response of the entire body to stress or infection.

4. *Strange, Rare, and Peculiar Symptoms.* Strange, rare, and peculiar symptoms are symptoms that are unique. Crawling sensations over the abdomen, cold sensations over the forehead, great thirst but for only sips at a time are examples. Strange, rare, and peculiar symptoms are the *most* important in selecting a homeopathic remedy, though, as the name implies, they are only rarely experienced and thus rarely found.

In determining a diagnosis and treatment, conventional physicians place the most emphasis on common symptoms; for homeopaths, these symptoms are the least important. This is simply because common symptoms do not help establish the uniqueness of a person's symptoms, and an individualized homeopathic remedy cannot be prescribed based on generalized symptoms. While conventional physicians try to fit a child into a specific diagnostic category, homeopaths try to determine how an individual child experiences an individual type of influenza, headache, or sore throat.

The ultimate effectiveness of a homeopathic medicine derives from matching the unique symptoms of the sick person with the unique symptoms a substance is known to cause. Because of this, parents should carefully assess which symptoms their child is experiencing that are idiosyncratic.

Homeopaths constantly confirm what most parents already know: that their child is unique. Although each child will have some symptoms that will be similar to those of other children, each will also have a distinct pattern of physical and psychological symptoms that is unique to that child alone.

For example, two children can both be suffering from a sore throat, but while your child will experience relief from sucking on an ice cube, your neighbor's child will get relief from sipping hot drinks. Your child may experience a head-ache with his sore throat, while your neighbor's child will have a cough. Your child may be lethargic, while the neighbor's child may be irritable.

Because distinctive symptoms help a homeopath find the individualized homeopathic medicine, the strange, rare, and peculiar symptoms are the most important in selecting a remedy. Since such symptoms are rare, however, homeopaths more commonly base their selection on the general symptoms. They then take into account the local symptoms. However, local symptoms merit more importance when they are severe or intense. In such instances the medicine chosen is known to treat these primary symptoms.

To summarize, the most important symptoms have one or more of the following characteristics:

- they are strange, rare, or peculiar;
- they are general symptoms (those that affect the whole body);
- they are intense symptoms.

An important point to clarify is that although homeopaths carefully evaluate the symptoms of a sick person, this doesn't mean that homeopathic treatment is *symptomatic*. Homeopaths don't treat symptoms; they simply *use* symptoms to determine which homeopathic medicine will most effectively trigger the body's healing response.

TAKING THE CHILD'S CASE

In order to determine what characteristic symptoms your child has, you have to know what questions to ask. Not only do you need to know where your child feels pain but also what the pain feels like, what things make it better or worse, and what other symptoms he is experiencing.

A useful trick to elicit this information is to avoid asking *yes* or *no* questions. Pose open-ended questions instead; your child is then free to discuss and describe his symptoms in greater detail. But don't make them leading questions: don't ask your son if his head hurts at night, ask him *when* does his head hurt. Rather than ask your daughter if her throat feels better when she drinks cold water, ask her if there is anything that relieves her throat pain.

Anything your child experiences which is different from what he normally does is worthy of attention. For instance, if your child is normally very energetic in the morning but now has the flu and is slow to get up, this symptom is more important than if your child is always slow to rise. If your child is normally slow to rise in the morning and feels the same way during a bout of the flu, clearly this symptom is not as important.

If your child's symptoms are considerably different from other children of the same age, this is also important. For instance, if a child is experiencing an aversion to sweets, this symptom is unusual and worth considering carefully.

Finding out an infant's symptoms is more difficult, but parents quickly become experts in noticing subtle but obvious behavior changes that may elude others. Sometimes it is necessary to experiment to find out how babies react to changes in their environment. You can open a window to see if the baby is irritated or relieved by it. You can uncover her to see if she cries, actively searches for her covers, or simply doesn't notice any change. You can give her cold and warm drinks to observe if she prefers one or the other. By making a sudden noise you can determine if she is easily startled.

Simple observation reveals much too. Is his pillow wet from sweat or salivation? Is he burrowing his head into the pillow, or is he trying to apply pressure to the front or back part of his head? Does he throw off his covers or stick his feet out? Is he lethargic or restless?

KEY LOCAL SYMPTOMS

Here are some questions that you can either ask yourself when treating an infant, or your child if he is old enough to answer. Many initial questions are open-ended so that the child can express what most concerns him.

What hurts the most?

Where does it hurt and what does it feel like?
Encourage your child to be specific about the pain's location and to describe what it feels like in as much detail as possible.

Did the symptom start slowly or come on rapidly?

Did the symptom start within 24 hours of doing something specific or feeling something unusual?

Sometimes children get ill after being exposed to cold air, a draft, being wet, or overheated because of the weather or over-exertion. Sometimes ailments begin after an emotional experience, most commonly anger, fear, grief, depression, anxiety, being startled, or jealousy. (Although children rarely connect emotional states with physical symptoms, parents, teachers, and other adults around them often notice these connections which can help you find the correct homeopathic medicine.)

MODALITIES

Various factors make a symptom better or worse, or they make a child feel better or worse: such factors are called *modalities*. A modality is simply something that either aggravates or relieves the child. A child's local symptom or general health may be better or worse at a certain time of the day, because of temperature or weather, or because of eating or drinking something. For example, a child's cough may be aggravated by heat: the aggravation from heat is the modality of the cough. Or, something may relieve one symptom but aggravate another. For instance, drinking cold drinks may relieve a sore throat but may aggravate digestive symptoms. Cold air may be irritating, but it may relieve a specific local symptom like a headache. Make certain to check these factors, since they are important in choosing the correct remedy.

TIME
Is there any time at which the pain is better or worse? See if your child's symptoms are better or worse on waking, during morning, afternoon, evening, night, before or after midnight, or at any particular hour.

TEMPERATURE AND WEATHER
Is there any temperature or weather condition that either aggravates or relieves symptoms? The child may either seek or be averse to cool rooms, warm rooms, stuffy rooms, the heat of a bed, the heat of a stove, the heat of the sun, open air, or drafts. Does the child open a window to get more fresh air or does he close a window because he is cold? The child may be affected by hot, cold, wet, dry, or stormy weather; wind, fog, snow, or changes in the weather. How much clothing does the child choose to wear?

BATHING
Does hot or cold bathing either aggravate or relieve any symptoms? If a child normally hates bathing but enjoys it during an illness, this may be important. Sometimes, however, the child may simply like a hot bath because he is chilly.

REST OR MOTION
Does rest or motion either aggravate or relieve any symptoms? Determine how the child is affected by slow or rapid motion, ascending or descending, initial motion or continued motion

(during and after), exertion (during and after), or passive motion (traveling in a car, boat, or plane).

Position
Are there positions that either aggravate or relieve any symptom? The child may be affected by standing, sitting, lying down, lying on the left or right side, lying on the back or stomach, lying on the painful or painless side, lying flat or lying with the head propped up, or lying in a fetal position.

External Stimuli
How is the child affected by touch (hard or soft), pressure, rubbing, noise, light, or odors? Whatever external stimuli affect the child's health can be important, especially if the child doesn't normally experience this hypersensitivity.

Eating or Drinking
Do any foods or drinks either aggravate or relieve any symptom? Determine if the child is affected by hot or cold food or drink, by swallowing, or by eating or drinking something specific. The most common foods to which children react are milk, bread, meat, pork, butter and fats, eggs, fish, fruit, onions, oysters, pastries, ice cream, potatoes, salt, spicy foods, and sweets.

Sleep
How does sleep affect the symptoms, and how do the symptoms affect sleep? Often symptoms in children are noticeably worse at night. Sometimes symptoms are worse before sleep, while other symptoms are worse during sleep.

Urination or Defecation
Are any symptoms better or worse before, during, or after urinating or defecating?

Sweat
Are any symptoms better or worse during or after a sweat? Some children feel relieved after sweating, while others feel lethargic afterward.

GENERAL SYMPTOMS

Appetite
Is there any food or drink that the child particularly craves or is averse to? Is the child always hungry? Rarely hungry? Does she eat slowly or rapidly? Specifically inquire if the child craves or detests milk, bread, meat, pork, butter and fats, eggs, fish, fruit, onions, oysters, pastries, ice cream, potatoes, salt, spicy foods, and sweets. Note that it is not a symptom if your child simply likes or doesn't like a particular food; only if there is an actual craving or an aversion does this become a symptom. Make certain to distinguish between those foods that only irritate your child from those that your child detests. Changes in a child's appetite during an acute illness are more important than the child's normal cravings or aversions.

Thirst
Does the child crave or detest hot or cold drinks? Does he take gulps or sips? Is he always thirsty or seldom thirsty?

Sleep
Is the child able to fall asleep and stay asleep? What position does she prefer? Does she wake up refreshed?

Sweat
Describe the child's sweating patterns. Do individual parts or does the whole body sweat excessively? Does the child sweat more on covered or uncovered parts of the body? Is there a characteristic odor to the sweat?

PSYCHOLOGICAL SYMPTOMS

Describe your child's psychological state just prior to and then during the illness. Is he fearful or anxious, depressed or irritable? Angry, obstinate, or easily offended? Get specific. If your child is fearful, what specific fears does she have? The dark, being alone, monsters, animals, heights, the future? If your child is sad, does he cry or try to hold it in? If he cries, does he cry quietly or does he sob? Is she irritable, or is anger a more accurate description? Enraged? Are her moods steady or do they shift frequently?

Is your child lethargic or restless? Easily startled? Does she prefer being alone, or being with family and friends? Does she want an audience?

Does he like sympathy, or is he irritated by being consoled? Is his room messier or cleaner than normal?

When irritated during illness, does your child hit others or throw things? Is he malicious or mischievous? Is he impulsive or overly controlled?

~

CHOOSING THE CORRECT HOMEOPATHIC MEDICINE

Finding the correct homeopathic medicine is like trying to match two similar puzzles. How does this work? Each symptom your child experiences is like a piece of a puzzle; the second puzzle has pieces which represent each symptom that a medicine is known to cure. The trick is to find the two similar puzzles.

While you ask your child or yourself questions about his symptoms, write down what is said. Homeopaths commonly use a system of underlining to help them assess the case. Underline those symptoms that are *unique* (strange, rare, or peculiar) or that are *intense*. Use more underlines depending upon the degree that the symptom is unique or intense (three underlines signifies a unique or very intense symptom; two underlines signifies a rare or intense one; one underline signifies a somewhat unusual or more-than-mild symptom; no underlining signifies symptoms that are noticeable but mild).

Extra underlining should sometimes be considered when children *spontaneously* describe symptoms, since such symptoms are often deeply felt.

Also remember that symptoms that affect *the whole child* (the general symptoms) are more important than local symptoms.

Use part 3 to help you find the most commonly given remedies for a specific condition. Do not only read the information presented under your child's ailment; look also to see if any of the medicines that may potentially fit your child's symptoms are in part 4. If so, read about the general characteristics of this medicine to see if the overall pattern of symptoms fits your child's.

Sometimes it will be difficult to determine which remedy is most appropriate because one medicine will fit some symptoms but not others, while another medicine will fit other symptoms but still not fit all of them.

You will only very rarely find a remedy that fits all of your child's symptoms. Most often there are some symptoms that your child is experiencing that are different in one way or another from one or more medicines. Place more emphasis on the general symptoms and on those symptoms that are particularly intense.

If it is still difficult to determine which remedy to choose, see if one of the medicines you are considering in part 3 is listed in all capital letters. These are the remedies most commonly indicated for that specific condition. Try this remedy first.

If the two remedies you are considering are both listed in capital letters or both in regular type, consider reviewing your child's symptoms one more time to see if you can discover anything new. Reread the general characteristics for each remedy in part 4 (if they are included there). Often the answer will become more clear after getting more detailed information about the potential remedies.

If you still aren't certain, look up the medicines you are

considering in Boericke's *Pocket Manual of Materia Medica with Repertory* or another *materia medica*. You might even try finding the correct remedy by using one of the computer software programs now available. (Although most homeopathic software programs have been developed for the practicing homeopath and are sophisticated and expensive, there is now at least one homeopathic software program that is easy for anyone to use. For more details, write to Homeopathic Educational Services, listed in the Resources section.)

If the answer still isn't clear, consider delaying the use of a homeopathic medicine until you are more confident. Or you may want to consult with a homeopath.

If, on the other hand, you decide to just use that famous parental intuition, you needn't worry too much.

Even if you give the wrong medicine, most often nothing happens. However, sometimes the wrong medicine is close enough to being the right remedy that it provides some benefit—but usually not enough to promote a full cure. These close, but not perfect, prescriptions can fool even experienced homeopaths. The following guidelines for choosing the correct potency and dose will help you determine when to continue giving a remedy and when to choose another medicine.

CHOOSING THE CORRECT POTENCY AND DOSE

The word *potency* refers to the number of times a medicine is potentized (the process of dilution and shaking, discussed in part 1). Homeopaths have discovered that the more a medicine is potentized, the faster and deeper it acts and the fewer doses of it are generally required for treatment.

The low potency medicines are those in the range of 3x–12x (*x* describing the number of times the medicine was diluted 1:10) or 3c–12c (*c* referring to the number of times it was diluted 1:100). Medium potency medicines are the 30x or 30c potencies, and higher potency medicines are the 200x, 200c, 1m (*m* is the Roman numeral of 1,000, thus this potency was diluted 1:100 1,000 times), 10m, 50m, and higher.

Some people who are new to homeopathy fret about which potency of a medicine to give. Such anxiety is needless. It is generally recognized in homeopathy that the choice of the correct medicine is significantly more important than the correct potency. Giving the incorrect potency will generally still promote healing, albeit slightly slower healing. It is likewise unnecessary to worry about whether to give an *x* or a *c* potency. They are both very similar in action, though the *c* potencies are considered slightly more powerful and therefore require slightly more precision in prescribing.

The word *dose* refers to the number of times a medicine is taken. The more intense a person's symptoms, the more frequent should be the dose, though the response to treatment also directly affects dosage. (You should slow down or stop taking the medicine as healing takes place.)

Determining the correct dose is important because in infrequent instances excessive dosages can lead to a proving (the experience of symptoms caused by the overdose). However, only rarely will a child experience a proving, and even in such cases, the symptoms dissipate shortly after the remedy is stopped.

Here are nine general rules for helping you determine the frequency of doses and level of potency of a homeopathy medicine.

1. *The basic rule in prescribing homeopathic medicines is to give as few doses as possible but as much as is necessary.* In acute disease a child's body usually needs repetition of a homeopathic remedy to continue to catalyze a healing response. However, because homeopathic medicines stimulate the body's own defenses (so that it can heal itself), it is

not always necessary to give continual doses of the medicines. Observe the child's symptoms. If the child is cured or even significantly better after only one or two doses, stop giving the remedy. If, however, the child has improved a little after several doses but is still sick, continue to give the remedy, unless it is now clear to you that another medicine is indicated. Do not, however, simply continue to give a remedy that doesn't seem to be working. Remember, homeopathic medicines are not vitamins; they are medicines that, when accurately prescribed, catalyze the body's own healing process. They are not necessarily made more effective by taking more doses of them.

2. *For people who are relatively new to homeopathy, it is recommended to use the 6th, 12th, or 30th potency (usually described as 6x or 6c, 12x or 12c, 30x or 30c).* The dose commonly recommended when using the 6th, 12th, or 30th potency is three to six times a day, depending upon the intensity of the symptoms. However, during the first day of a high fever or other inflammatory condition, you may need to give the remedy every hour or every other hour during the first twenty-four-hour period of the illness. Typically, some degree of relief from an acute problem is usually observed after a night's rest. Chronic or recurring complaints take longer and may require constitutional care from a professional homeopath.

3. *It is generally recommended not to use any potencies higher than the 30th unless you are very familiar with homeopathic philosophy, methodology, and materia medica.* Although higher potencies have a smaller material dose of the substance, homeopaths usually find that they are actually

stronger than the less potentized doses. These higher potencies sometimes cause a healing crisis—that is, a temporary worsening of symptoms prior to a deep cure. Practitioners trained in homeopathy are more likely to know when worsening of symptoms is really a healing crisis or if it simply represents the child becoming more ill.

4. *The more severe symptoms a child experiences, the more frequent repetition of a remedy is necessary.* For high fevers, intense inflammatory conditions, or strong pain, you may need to give the remedy every hour or every other hour. For mild symptoms, it is common to give a remedy three or four times in a day. Usually you can give the 6th or 12th potency for up to a week, while the 30th potency is not commonly given for more than three days at a time.

5. *The more intense the symptoms, the higher the potency is recommended.* If your child's symptoms are intense, as opposed to mild or simply persistent, it is recommended to use the 30th potency; it will act faster and deeper than the 6th potency.

6. *Generally, the more confident you are in the selection of your remedy, especially if the medicine matches the general symptoms, the higher the potency should be used.* Using the 30th potency requires more precision in prescribing than using the 6th or the 12th. The higher the potency used, the closer to the bull's eye the remedy should be.

7. *Allow enough time for the remedy to act before changing to another remedy.* Homeopathic medicines sometimes act very rapidly, but they can also act slowly. Sometimes a child may still be sick after taking a remedy for a couple of days, though some

key symptoms have improved. It is important to avoid changing remedies while the child is in the process of improvement. If, however, the child is having intense symptoms and there is *no* improvement after twenty-four hours, a new remedy should be considered. If the child has mild symptoms, wait at least thirty-six to forty-eight hours before considering a new remedy. (One important exception to this rule is if your child develops new symptoms and you are now confident that another remedy is more accurate; then you can consider switching remedies.)

8. *Try to avoid giving several remedies per episode of illness.* Some parents are impatient and expect a homeopathic medicine or any medicine to immediately cure their child. Try to avoid switching medicines too quickly or too often. If you give too many different remedies in an episode of illness, you are not giving the remedies enough time to act. In rare instances it is possible to antidote the correct remedy by giving another medicine too soon. Do not give more than three or four medicines per episode; ideally, you should use just one or two.

9. *You can stop giving the remedy once you notice that your child is considerably better.* Although some practitioners or parents give additional doses of a remedy when a child still has minor symptoms, the general rule in homeopathy is to use as few doses as possible. If a medicine has obviously provided considerable benefit, the child's body will be able to complete the healing. In cases when this doesn't happen, either a couple more doses of the original remedy is indicated, or a new medicine can be chosen that fits the present symptoms.

HOW TO GIVE HOMEOPATHIC MEDICINES

Homeopathic medicines usually come in pellet form, most often in a lactose (milk sugar) or sucrose base. Sometimes these pellets are very small, looking almost like cake sprinkles (these are called #10 pellets); sometime they come in larger spherical globules (#35 pellets); and sometimes in conventional aspirin-like pill form. Some companies place their medications in liquid—usually distilled water that is preserved with alcohol. There is no real difference in quality or effect between these various forms.

The sweet taste of the lactose or sucrose-based remedies makes them very palatable for infants and children. Some parents crush the globules or pills when giving them to infants to make certain they will not choke on them.

The medicine should be placed under the tongue so that it can dissolve slowly—though sucking on the remedy and then chewing it works too. It is not recommended to wash down the medicine with water.

It is generally advised to take either 5–10 of the cake sprinkle pellets per dose, 2–4 of the spherical globules, or 1–2 of the pills. Directions are always provided on the bottle.

When possible, avoid handling a remedy with your hands. It is best to place the remedy into the cap of the bottle and then pour or place the remedy in the child's mouth. If you want to crush a remedy to make it easier for an infant to take, use clean and dry silverware, and then clean it thoroughly afterward to remove all traces of the remedy.

Ideally, the child should not eat, drink (except water), brush teeth, chew gum, or take cough drops for fifteen minutes before or after taking a homeopathic remedy—though this general rule can be broken if necessary. If, for instance, a child injures herself shortly after eating a meal, do not hesitate to give her a medicine at that point.

One of the clear benefits of homeopathic medicines is

their safety. If an infant or child accidentally ate an entire bottle of a homeopathic medicine, there is generally nothing to worry about. There are so few, if any, molecules of the medicine that no effects would result. The child would be getting a greater dose of lactose or sucrose than of any medicinal substance. The only time a problem could happen is if an unsupervised infant or child took a couple of pellets every hour for several days. Even in this worst-case scenario, the child would experience a proving of the substance, and whatever symptoms might emerge will stop shortly after the last dose.

WHAT TO AVOID WHILE TAKING A HOMEOPATHIC MEDICINE

Homeopaths have found that certain things can potentially act as an antidote to a homeopathic medicine. Although no substance acts upon a remedy in this way in *every* instance, it is generally recommended for your child to avoid the following during the days he is taking homeopathic medicines:

- Camphor and camphorated products (commonly found in various lip balms and muscle-relaxing creams such as Ben Gay, Vick's Heet, Campho-Phenique, Tiger Balm, and Noxzema);

- Mint or mentholated products (commonly found in mouthwashes, cough drops, and toothpastes);

- Electric blankets (it is thought that electric blankets may disturb the body's nervous system and subtle physiological processes);

- Dental drilling or teeth cleaning (we do not understand how or why this has an effect, though it is theorized that dental drilling or cleaning strongly stimulates acupuncture points in the teeth and then neutralizes the actions of the remedy);

- Some allopathic drugs, especially steroidal drugs such as cortisone and prednizone, can also act as an antidote to the action of a homeopathic medicine. Although most allopathic drugs do not do so, they do tend to alter the person's symptoms so that the correct homeopathic remedy cannot be found as easily.

Homeopaths sometimes find that coffee also has this effect, though this is rarely a problem for children.

HOW TO TAKE CARE OF YOUR HOMEOPATHIC MEDICINES

If homeopathic medicines are given proper care, they will remain potent for many decades—often longer. Here are some basic guidelines for keeping and storing them.

- Prevent exposure to long-term direct sunlight or other intense light;
- Avoid exposure to temperatures higher than 100 degrees;
- Keep separate from strong smelling odors, especially camphor, perfumes, and mothballs (it is generally recommended to not place them in medicine cabinets due to the presence of such odors, either past or present);
- Avoid potential contamination by quickly replacing the cap on the homeopathic bottle;
- Keep the medicine in the original container, though you can place several doses in folded-up sheets of clean paper so that you child can take them when away from home;

- If any medicine falls to the floor, it is best to throw it away rather than place it back in the bottle.

WHEN TO SEEK PROFESSIONAL HOMEOPATHIC CARE

This book focuses on the use of homeopathic medicines in treating common *acute* conditions of your infant or child. Although homeopaths encourage parents to provide care for their family's acute ailments, they discourage efforts to treat *chronic* conditions at home.

Any symptom or syndrome that your child has repeatedly should be treated by a professional homeopath. Part 3 of this book describes some conditions which are sometimes chronic in nature. Although parents may try to treat their children for these conditions if a professional homeopath is not available, it is often worth traveling the necessary distance to find a good practitioner.

Parents should also seek conventional medical care for certain potentially dangerous conditions. Finding a good pediatrician who is open to and perhaps interested in homeopathy and other alternative medicines may be difficult but is worth the effort. Because a growing number of professional homeopaths are also medical doctors, naturopathic physicians, or some other licensed medical professional, you receive the best of both worlds by seeking their care.

There are several readily available books that can help you determine when your child's symptoms are serious enough to warrant medical attention: *Care for Your Baby and Your Child* edited by Steven Shelov and *Dr. Spock's Baby and Child Care* by Benjamin Spock and Michael Rothenberg; both include this important medical information.

To find a professional homeopath, write or call Homeopathic Educational Services or any of the homeopathic organizations listed in the Resources section.

The benefits that good professional homeopathic care can offer a child's health should not be underestimated. Such care can successfully heal chronic ailments, reduce the severity and frequency of acute conditions, and prevent various diseases. At the same time, there are substantial benefits readily available to anyone armed with the information in this book. You will be able to successfully treat at home a wide variety of acute ailments and injuries quickly.

Perhaps the best care of all is a collaborative model of healing, in which parents learn to treat their children for common acute conditions and seek professional homeopathic care for more serious or chronic ailments. Such intelligent and effective health care will be of long-lasting benefit to your child.

PART 3

Common Ailments
of Children

~

Most parents will probably begin reading this part of the book after their child is already ill. The child is now frantically demanding help. Parents new to homeopathy will be surprised, even amazed, at how effective homeopathic medicines can be in giving their child this help.

Look up your child's illness in this section first and read the descriptions of *all* the medicines listed under the ailment. Even after you find a remedy that seems to match your child's symptoms, continue reading the descriptions of the other medicines; you may find a remedy that matches your child's symptoms even more closely.

To find the best remedy for your child, you can complement the information in part 3 with the more detailed information in part 4, which discusses the general characteristics of those homeopathic medicines, underlined in part 3, which are the most useful for your home pharmacy. If you have difficulty figuring out which medicine to use, even after reviewing the more detailed information in part 4, give your child the medicine that appears in all capital letters. These medicines have the best track record of success in treating children with that complaint.

Most of the homeopathic manufacturers sell homeopathic medicine kits which include between twenty-five to fifty remedies. These kits are sold at significant discounts, often half the price of purchasing the medicines individually. Because children have a tendency to become ill at night, especially late at night, it can be a great relief to have a homeopathic medicine kit on hand. Appendix II lists sources of homeopathic medicine and homeopathic kits.

To obtain even more detailed information about a homeopathic medicine described in this book, look through one of the homeopathic *materia medicas* listed in the bibliography.

It may be helpful for parents to know that although the information provided in this book is directed toward children's ailments, these same medicines are equally effective in similar dosages for the same illnesses in adults. The pronouns *he* and *she* are used interchangeably throughout this part of the book. Their use does not mean that a specific medicine should only be used to treat a boy or a girl, but that it can be used to treat either as long as the symptoms match.

How to Use this Section

CAPITAL LETTERS = the most commonly used medicines for that particular ailment.

<u>Underlined medicines</u> = those medicines discussed in more detail in part 4.

ALLERGIES (RESPIRATORY)
See also Asthma, Hives, Indigestion,
or the individual symptom of the allergy.

Homeopathic medicines are often effective in treating the acute symptoms of allergies, though professional constitutional care is usually necessary to achieve a deeper cure of the chronic allergic state.

<u>ALLIUM CEPA</u>: Children who will benefit from *Allium cepa* experience a profuse, watery, burning nasal discharge which is worse in a warm room and better in the open air. They have

ALLERGIES

reddened eyes with bland (non-burning) tears and want to rub their eyes frequently. There is a raw feeling in the nose with a tingling sensation as well as violent sneezing. A frontal congestive headache may go along with their allergy symptoms. These symptoms tend to worsen after damp winds.

Ambrosia: This is the primary remedy for hay fever after exposure to ragweed (*Ambrosia* is a homeopathic dose of ragweed). These children have a watery nasal discharge, and tearing, itchy eyes. They may also have an irritated throat and asthmatic breathing.

Apis: Swelling of the throat which is worse with heat is a common allergic reaction of these children. They cannot stand anything around their necks and have a sense of constriction in their chests. There may be hives and puffiness around the face, swollen eyelids, and swelling under the eyes. The child sometimes suffers from intolerable itching, especially at night in bed, and his skin may feel swollen, tense, tight, and hypertensive to touch.

ARSENICUM: Symptoms are burning tears and nasal discharge, often worse on the right side. The symptoms are worse after midnight. The child tosses and turns in bed and becomes very anxious during breathing difficulties. He is very chilly and feels better in a warm room. He's very thirsty but only takes sips at a time. He is also sensitive to light, sneezes violently, and may breathe asthmatically.

EUPHRASIA: Children who need *Euphrasia* have the opposite symptoms as those who need *Allium cepa:* they have profuse burning tears and a bland nasal discharge. Their eyes water so much they look like they are constantly crying. Their eyes and cheeks become red from the burning tears. The eye symptoms are worse in the open air; the nasal discharge is worse at night, when lying down, and in windy weather.

Kali bic: When children with an allergy have a thick, gluey, stringy, yellow nasal discharge, this medicine is invaluable.

ALLERGIES

They may also have post-nasal drip with sticky mucus, and pain at the root of the nose which feels better when pressure is applied. The child may constantly want to blow his nose. The discharge, along with the sneezing, is worse from exposure to cold or in the open air. The child may also have a cough at the same time, or a swollen throat which is relieved by warm liquids.

Natrum mur: This remedy is most often given to children who get hay fever attacks every spring and fall and who seem to develop their symptoms after an emotional experience, especially grief. Death, divorce, unrequited love, or homesickness often create feelings that are not fully expressed, eventually leading to various physical complaints; this medicine helps. These children also sneeze frequently, have a profuse watery discharge from their noses and eyes, and lose their senses of taste and smell. Eventually, the nasal discharge may lead to chronic nasal congestion and thick white mucus. The symptoms are worse in the morning, when the child usually coughs up much mucus. Dry and cracked lips or a cold sore may accompany the hay fever symptoms.

<u>NUX VOMICA</u>: These children are irritable and chilly and tend to have steady nasal discharges during the day and are congested at night. Their symptoms tend to be worse indoors and better in the open air. They are sensitive to the cold and to being uncovered. There may be frequent sneezing. The symptoms sometimes begin after the child has been irritated or fatigued.

<u>PULSATILLA</u>: These children have runny noses during the day and are congested at night. Their congestion is worse in a warm room, during hot weather, or while lying down, and is relieved by cool rooms, open air, or by cool applications. The roof of the child's mouth itches at night. She is moody and impressionable. She seems to never be thirsty. *Pulsatilla* is more commonly given to girls than to boys, though personality, not

gender, determines its use. If the child is moody, impressionable, and craves sympathy consider this medicine.

SABADILLA: These children feel worse in the cold air. They sneeze spasmodically, have itchy, runny noses, and red, runny eyes. The child may also get headaches in her forehead and feel a lump in her throat with a constant desire to swallow. Like a child that responds well to *Pulsatilla* she will have a dry throat but not be thirsty. She seems to always be chilly.

<u>Sulphur</u>: This child has his hay fever in the summer and the condition is aggravated by heat and sun. He has a stuffed-up nose when indoors and a constantly runny nose when outdoors. The nose and eyes are red, and the nasal discharge burns. As the condition develops, the nasal discharge begins to smell bad. The allergy can develop into asthma, especially after exertion.

Wyethia: This child has an irritable itching behind her nose or in the roof of her mouth. She also has a tickling sensation that gives her a dry, hacking cough. Her throat feels swollen, and she has a constant desire to swallow saliva but has difficulty swallowing.

ANGER

Homeopathic medicines can often treat the acute symptoms of anger—though professional constitutional care is usually necessary for a deeper level of cure. Professional psychological care might also be considered when a child has recurrent bouts of anger. (See "General Characteristics" under each remedy in part 4 for more detailed information.)

<u>Bryonia</u>: This is "the grumpy bear" remedy: these children are irritable and want to be left alone. They will grumble or

snap, if necessary, to keep others away. They tend to get digestive, respiratory, or headache symptoms after a bout of anger.

CHAMOMILLA: Children who need *Chamomilla* "cannot bear it"—the pain, other people, themselves, anything; not even to be looked at or spoken to. They demand things but then discard them. The only way to provide relief, albeit temporary relief, is to rock or carry the child. This passive motion is soothing; however, shortly after putting the child down, the screaming and crying often returns. He is tempermental, throws things, is impatient, and may even bang his head against a wall. Various physical symptoms may arise after an emotional outburst, though it is as likely that physical symptoms will begin first and then lead to hyperirritability.

COLOCYNTHIS: These children complain constantly. Other than this complaining, they are disinclined to talk to people. They are irritable and impatient, and are offended at everything. They usually develop vomiting, diarrhea, or colic during or after their bouts of anger.

IGNATIA: Children who need *Ignatia* don't express their emotions, nor do they stick up for themselves when they have been hurt. They hold in their anger, grief, or fear, and pretend that everything is OK. They may expose this internal anxiety by trembling. They sigh frequently. Finally, their inner turmoil is expressed through hysteria. Children who will be helped by *Ignatia* do not get angry and stay angry; nor are they violent. They generally feel misunderstood and reject sympathy. Their moods are changeable: laughter and tears alternate or mingle; they may be very angry and then suddenly be remorseful and repentant; they may be rude and rebellious, and then become docile.

NUX VOMICA: This child throws tantrums and fends off anyone who tries to stop him from doing what he wants to do. He thrives on rebellion. He is competitive and gets angry at anyone who might make him lose. He is irritable and fault-

ANGER

finding. He tends to have digestive symptoms (constipation, gas, acid indigestion) or difficulty sleeping after a bout of anger.

Stramonium: When a child is out of control with rage, this medicine should be considered. The child becomes wild and has delusions: she hears voices and may claim to see ghosts, animals, or the Devil. She believes that she has been abandoned, or feels that she is falling. She is talkative and may curse loudly or often. Some children who need this medicine develop a stutter.

<u>STAPHYSAGRIA</u>: This remedy is for the child that suppresses his anger and silently stews about his problem. He can, however, only repress his feelings for so long—eventually, he explodes in rage. He trembles, loses his voice, throws things, demands something but then refuses it once it's offered. He can't concentrate, becomes exhausted, and has insomnia. These children are quite distinct from children who benefit from *Chamomilla* (who are too irritable to hold anything inside), or those who are helped by *Ignatia* (who have more frequent swings of emotion as well as noticeable sighing). *Staphysagria* is for children who are sensitive to the least offense—sometimes every word said to them is taken the wrong way. If they finally explode, they tend to feel bad about it afterward. These children have their physical ailments either shortly after they suppress their anger or just after they express it. *Staphysagria* is a common remedy for children who have been abused physically or sexually.

ANXIETY,
ailments from or with

Homeopathic medicines can often treat the acute symptoms of anxiety, though professional constitutional care is usually necessary for the deeper cure of a chronic condition. Professional psychological help may be essential when a child has recurrent bouts of anxiety. (See "General Characteristics" under each underlined remedy in part 4 for more detailed information.)

ACONITUM: A sense of panic and frantic impatience is felt by children who need this remedy. They have an intangible but real fear that something awful may happen. They may, for instance, feel that they are so sick that they are going to die. They are easily startled.

Argentum nit: This child tends to develop physical illness because of the anxiety he feels before a performance or examination. He is terrified that something will go wrong.

ARSENICUM: The motto of a child who needs this medicine might be "Anything worth doing is worth overdoing." This child is a perfectionist. She is fastidious, fussy about her appearance, and tidy, even when ill. She exaggerates her illness, acting more sick than she really is. She is unduly anxious—worried about almost everything, particularly when something is expected of her.

GELSEMIUM: This child is anxious before an examination, a competitive game, a speech, a performance, or any act that requires courage. He may get diarrhea or a headache from his anxiety. He shakes: his hands tremble when he lifts something; his feet tremble when he is sitting or walking; his tongue quivers when he sticks it out. Even his voice may tremble.

IGNATIA: A child who needs *Ignatia* doesn't express her emotions, and doesn't stick up for herself when she has been hurt. She holds in her feelings and pretends nothing is wrong. She may expose her anxiety by trembling; she sighs; finally, she explodes. She is upset by trifles and easily offended. *Ignatia* is also recommended for high-strung or sensitive children after they have been reprimanded. It's good for homesickness, too.

ANXIETY

Lycopodium: When ill, this child feels insecure and always wants someone around. He may not need someone at his bedside but someone must at least be in a room nearby. *Lycopodium* is effective for the bedwetting child who is very anxious, constantly worrying about what others think of him or fearful of trying anything new. Children helped by *Lycopodium* may be quite arrogant and bullying as a way to hide their deep insecurities. Evidence of this insecurity is a tendency to be easily embarrassed and a fear of failure. They may also have performance anxiety. Prior to the performance, the child tends to boast about this ability, and yet, once the performance approaches, he becomes increasingly insecure, though he does his best to hide it.

Natrum mur: These children tend to have a long-term emotional memory. Once they are hurt, they do not let go of the pain easily: they bear grudges and dwell on past problems. Death, divorce, lack of parental love, or homesickness may create anxiety which is unexpressed, eventually leading to various physical complaints. They are noticeably averse to sympathy and want to be left alone.

Phosphorus: This child is strongly influenced by others: if someone around him is worried about his health, then he becomes worried too; when others are hopeful, then he too will be hopeful. A child that responds to *Phosphorus* seeks company and affection. In particular, he wants sympathy. He is susceptible to certain typical fears: of the dark, of his disease, of thunder, of being alone, and of spiders. He may feel this fear in the pit of his stomach. He may tremble from the slightest cause, or become restless and fidget constantly.

Silicea: These children are very shy and have a fear of doing new things because they fear failure. Although they lack confidence, they are actually quite bright and usually do things well if they finish them. Children who need this remedy do not stand up for themselves, and wilt from their lack of grit

ANXIETY

unless they are given much encouragement. They are easily startled and easily irritated by little things. Sometimes little things upset them more than big things. They can be very stubborn, though they won't be aggressive or argumentative; instead, they will be pleasant as long as they can do it their own way.

∾

ASTHMA

Asthma is a potentially serious and even life-threatening condition. Infants and children with asthma should receive medical attention. Be aware that conventional drugs used for treating asthma, particularly steroids, can impair immune function and lead to more serious health problems. The following remedies can reduce the distress that an acute attack can create, but homeopathic constitutional care is necessary to achieve a lasting cure.

Aconitum: This remedy is very useful at the very beginning onset of asthmatic breathing. Noticeably present with the asthma are anxiety, fear, and restlessness.

Antimonium tart: The characteristic symptom of children who need this remedy is a rattling cough with an inability to expectorate mucus. Their condition sometimes starts after being angered or annoyed. They feel drowsy and feeble, and their symptoms are usually worse at 4:00 A.M. They may want to sit up rather than lie down because of difficulty breathing. Along with these breathing difficulties they are anxious, restless, and irritable. They feel chilly but can't stand stuffy, warm rooms and want cool rooms and open windows. This remedy is rarely given at the beginning of an illness.

ARSENICUM: Restlessness and anxiety are prominent. As the asthma continues, the child gets more and more frightened. His symptoms are worse from midnight to 2:00 A.M., and he tosses and turns in bed. His breathing is best when sitting erect. Despite his restlessness, he is tired and weak. He is chilly and feels better with warmth. He is thirsty but for only sips of water at a time.

Chamomilla: This remedy should be considered for asthma brought on by a tantrum. This child is impatient with her suffering. She has a hard, dry cough during sleep; difficulty breathing is relieved by bending her head backward, being in cold air, or drinking cold water.

IPECAC: There is persistent nausea with a loose cough and a rattling in the chest but an inability to expectorate. The child wheezes and has sticky mucus that is blood-streaked. Vomiting provides some relief of the child's symptoms because it helps to eliminate mucus. The symptoms are worse in hot, humid weather and are aggravated by the least motion. There is cold sweat on the child's extremities. They may also have difficulty sleeping, and will tend to salivate excessively.

Lobelia: This remedy is known to cure asthmatic breathing accompanied by nausea and vomiting. These children usually have prickling sensations all over, even on the fingers and toes; this precedes the asthma. The asthma is aggravated by exposure to cold. The child may feel weakness in the pit of the stomach and a sensation of a lump above the sternum (the chest bone).

Nux vomica: This remedy is good for treating asthma when the child feels full in the stomach, especially in the morning or after eating. He has asthma accompanied by choking, anxiety, pressure in the pit of the stomach, humming in the ears, quick pulse, and sweating. The child's attack is sometimes incited by hay fever. He feels he must loosen clothing around his waist. Emotionally, the child is more irritable than fearful.

PULSATILLA: The child has asthmatic breathing in warm or stuffy rooms, in warm weather, or after eating fatty or rich

ASTHMA

foods. She wants the windows open and to feel cool air. She is more apt to have breathing difficulties in the evening, especially after a meal. She craves sympathy and the company of others. She is very clingy and needy. She is highly impressionable: if parents are anxious about the child, the child becomes more anxious; if parents are confident in the child's ability to get healthy soon, the child will be soothed.

Sambucus: The child gets his asthma attack during sleep, commonly awakening him at 3:00 A.M. Breathing is obstructed when he lies down and is partially relieved when he sits up as he gasps for air. His breathing then improves, but is aggravated again when he lies back down to sleep. The child sweats profusely while awake but tends not to perspire during sleep.

Spongia: This remedy is known to be helpful for children with asthma who have a dry, barking, croupy cough. Their air passages are dry, sputum is absent, and their voices are hoarse. The asthma can be exacerbated by cold air, warm rooms, tobacco smoke, talking, lying with their heads low, drinking cold fluids, or eating sweets. The symptoms also tend to be worse in the early part of the night. Warm food or drinks, even in small doses, provide some relief, as does sitting up and leaning forward.

~

BACKACHE

Homeopathic medicines are effective for backaches, though massage and other physical therapies as well as therapeutic exercise can complement homeopathic care.

Arnica: Consider using this for children with a backache from injury or overuse of the back muscles.

Bryonia: The child has aching or stitching pain from the slightest motion. He feels better when he is motionless, though in extreme cases of backache he may still feel sore and bruised even when he is at rest. Firm pressure gives some relief.

HYPERICUM: When back pain of a sharp or shooting nature is caused by an injury—either a fall or blow to the back—this remedy should be considered. Another indication for its use is when the child's back pains are aggravated by lifting his arms. This remedy is invaluable for backaches in an athletic child whose spine is frequently under stress due to exercise.

Magnesia phos: This remedy is of immense value when a child has shooting or stitching pains in the back that are sensitive to touch and feel better with warm applications.

Nux vomica: If heaviness and stiffness of the neck is accompanied by digestive problems or a headache or both, this remedy should be given. It is also good for lower back pain accompanied by constipation. Symptoms are worse in the morning, after eating, and when the back is touched. The child has difficulty turning over in bed and has spasms aggravated by the slightest touch.

RHUS TOX: This remedy is considered the best medicine for lower back pain, especially when the pains are worse when the child first moves but lessen if he keeps moving. It is also good for similar pains between the shoulder blades or for a stiff neck. The symptoms of pain and stiffness are worse at night and first thing in the morning. They are sometimes worse in the cold and better in the heat. Back pain may be caused by overexertion, lifting heavy objects, or injury. The child may become stiff after getting wet or chilled.

~

BEDWETTING

A child who has stopped bedwetting but has begun to do so again should have a urine culture to rule out kidney disease.

BEDWETTING

Professional homeopathic care may be necessary to fully cure this problem, though the above medicines can provide some relief. Behavioral or psychological therapy may help too.

Belladonna: The child tends to dribble urine when he is cold or chilled. He may have burning pains along the length of the urethra during urination. He tends to have wild dreams and often dreams of urinating.

Causticum: Bedwetting is usually worse in the winter and better in the summer. Various fears accompany the child's bedwetting, especially fears that something bad will happen to him. He is afraid of going to bed in the dark. He tends to wet his pants when he coughs or sneezes or even laughs.

EQUISETUM: This remedy is for children who wet the bed for no apparent reason other than habit. Consider *Equisetum* when the child has no other obvious symptoms. Give it also when the child has wild dreams or nightmares when bedwetting. He tends to dream of crowds of people. This medicine is most often helpful in low potency (3 or 6).

Ferrum phos: This remedy is more effective for daytime pants-wetting, especially when the child feels the strongest urges to urinate while standing. The child's urge is less when he is lying down.

Kreosotum: Consider using for children who have such a sudden urge to urinate that they do not have enough time to get out of bed to go to the bathroom. These children tend to wet their beds during the first part of the night. Sometimes they will have dreams that they are urinating.

Lycopodium: This remedy is for the bedwetting child who constantly worries about what others think of him. He usually has fears of trying anything new. He is more prone to wet the bed if he sleeps in a warm or stuffy room. He prefers to sleep with the window open.

BEDWETTING

Pulsatilla: The child cannot lie on her back in bed without feeling the urge to urinate. *Pulsatilla* is also an effective remedy for bedwetting during or after the measles.

Sepia: The child wets the bed shortly after going to sleep or in the early evening. If you can help the child avoid wetting the bed before 10:00 P.M., it is likely that she will stay dry all night.

SULPHUR: The child sleeps with his feet sticking out or tosses off the covers. He wants open air, wakes up at 5:00 A.M., and has vivid dreams. (See "General Characteristics" in part 4 for more information about this type of child.)

BIRTH TRAUMA

ACONITUM: When the mother is very afraid of giving birth, this remedy can calm her. After birth, the infant may need this medicine as well to help reduce the fear it felt due to this anxious birth.

ARNICA: This is the primary medicine for the trauma of birth, and is recommended for both mother and infant. It is also good for the mother's muscle aches caused by straining during labor and helps to promote proper uterine contraction. It can also stop uterine bleeding during or after labor.

Hypericum: This remedy is for injuries to the head, spine, hands, or feet during birth or for nerve injuries during birth.

Natrum sulphur: Use for babies who develop persistent, chronic symptoms due to trauma to the head during labor.

STRAMONIUM: This medicine is the first to consider for infants who suffer from convulsions because of birth trauma. The infant wakes frequently at night and is terrified.

BIRTH TRAUMA

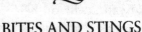

BITES AND STINGS

APIS: This medicine is good for red, inflamed insect bites which cause burning or stinging pain; symptoms are worse with heat or warm applications and are relieved by cold or cool applications.

Hypericum: Use *Hypericum* when a child develops sharp or shooting pains from a bite or sting.

LEDUM: This is the most common medicine for itching bites or stings from mosquitoes, bees, wasps, spiders, and rats. The itching from the bite or sting is relieved by cold applications and is sensitive to touch.

Staphysagria: Use for mosquito or other insect bites that itch excessively or create large welts.

BLACK EYE. See Eye Injuries.

BLADDER INFECTION
(Cystitis)

Recent research suggests that *any* child with a bladder infection should receive prompt medical attention to determine if there is a urinary tract defect.

Aconitum: This remedy should be considered at the first symptoms of a bladder infection. Urination is hot and painful and may even make the child scream. Typically, the child is very thirsty.

Berberis: If a child has a bladder infection in which he feels pain from any motion or jar, consider this remedy. The child feels burning and stitching pain during urination and feels aching in the bladder even when not urinating.

BLADDER INFECTION

CANTHARIS: This child has a sudden and frequent urge to urinate, and yet is only able to urinate a little at a time, with painful, drop-by-drop burning before, during, or after. She is restless and changes positions frequently. Her urine may have a reddish tint, suggesting blood in the urine.

Equisetum: The child feels a burning pain in the uretha toward the end of urination. She has a great desire to urinate, but can only pass a small amount at a time.

PULSATILLA: This remedy is indicated when cystitis starts after the child gets suddenly chilled during hot weather. She has a frequent urge to urinate, with pain before and during. She may also dribble urine after a cough, sneeze, or laugh. The child is moody and weepy. She craves affection and sympathy, and is averse to warm rooms and is not thirsty.

SARSPARILLA: The child feels unbearable pain at the end of urination, has difficulty urinating when sitting, and can only do so in dribbles. Sometimes he has a painful urge to urinate but is unable to do so. The child finds that it is easier and less painful to urinate while standing.

STAPHYSAGRIA: This remedy should be considered when a child gets a bladder infection after sexual or physical abuse or after humiliation or suppressing anger. The child has burning pains in the urethra even when not urinating and has a frequent desire to urinate.

BLEEDING

Homeopathic medicines, when correctly prescribed, can stop bleeding immediately. To stop the bleeding is of primary importance in first aid; do all that you can with pressure or ice as well. Medical care should be sought if there is much blood

BLEEDING

loss. Internal bleeding should receive immediate medical attention.

Aconitum: This is the first remedy to consider when there is great restlessness, anxiety, and fear along with the bleeding.

ARNICA: Give this remedy for the initial shock and trauma that the child experiences from an injury. It is very effective for both internal or external bleeding.

CALENDULA: External application of *Calendula* reduces and stops bleeding and prevents infection. It is also good for dental hemorrhages; have the child rinse her mouth with *Calendula* tincture.

HAMAMELIS: When a child bleeds profusely from a cut or wound, this remedy, like *Arnica,* often acts immediately. It is the first remedy to consider for profuse bleeding from the nose. (*Phosphorus* is the second remedy to consider.) If, during the bleeding or after it stops, there is intense soreness of the injured part this medicine can quickly soothe it. It is also indicated when the white part of a child's eye becomes bright red due to the breaking of a blood vessel. Although hemorrhoids are not very common in children, *Hamamelis* is useful for children who get them, especially for bleeding hemorrhoids.

Ipecac: If a child gets frequent nosebleeds of bright red blood, consider this medicine. It's also invaluable for a child who experiences any type of bleeding along with nausea, faintness, or air hunger (difficulty taking a deep breath, sometimes needing others to fan him to help him get oxygen).

Phosphorus: The child gets frequent nosebleeds and fits the *Phosphorus* constitution. (See "General Characteristics" in part 4.) This is also a primary remedy for dental hemorrhage.

BLEEDING

BOILS

BELLADONNA: These children have hot, painful and shiny red boils. This remedy is usually most effective when given before pus forms.

HEPAR SULPHUR: When a boil is extremely sensitive to touch, this medicine is often very effective. There is often a sensation as though there was a stick under the skin. This remedy is also effective for any small injury which turns into a boil.

SILICEA: This remedy is for a child who develops a boil at the slightest scratch.

Sulphur: Consider *Sulphur* when a child gets reddened hot boils—sometimes in crops—or boils that tend to return shortly after previous ones have disappeared. There is often a red or purplish circle around the eruption. These boils frequently form on the buttocks. Classically, these children have dry, scaly, dirty-looking skin.

BONE INJURIES

These medicines should be taken on the way to the doctor's office and again after a splint has been applied. It is unnecessary to take the medicine for more than fourteen days.

Arnica: This medicine should be taken immediately after a bone injury for the shock.

Bryonia: *Bryonia* is the first remedy to consider for fractured ribs. Also, give *Bryonia* if the pain of a fracture or other bone injury persists even though *Arnica, Symphytum*, and *Calcarea phos* have been given.

BONE INJURIES

Calcarea phos: This remedy should be considered after giving *Symphytum* when a fracture is slow to heal.

RUTA: Injuries to the periosteum (the covering around the bone) and to the knee, shin, or elbow should be treated with *Ruta.*

SYMPHYTUM: This is the primary remedy to speed the healing of bones or for injuries to the cheekbone or bones around the eye.

BONE PAINS
See Growing Pains.

BRONCHITIS
See Cough.

BRUISES

ARNICA: This is the best remedy for the shock of injury. It also helps the body absorb the blood under the skin. In addition to internal doses, external applications of *Arnica* gel, spray, or ointment should be used—but only when the skin has not been broken.

Bellis perennis: This remedy is primarily used for injuries to the internal organs or to the breast.

HYPERICUM: Used for injuries to the nerves or to parts of the body richly supplied with nerves (back, hands, feet).

Ledum: This remedy reduces the black-and-blue discoloration when *Arnica* is not working well enough. It is the primary remedy for a black eye and for injuries from a blow from firm objects. It is the best remedy for wounds that are cold to the touch and made worse by warmth, especially the warmth of bed. Usually, the wound is very sensitive to touch.

BRUISES

Ruta: For injuries to the periosteum (the bone covering) or for injuries to the knee, shin bone, and elbow. It is also good for bruises that create a hard nodule under the skin.

SYMPHYTUM: Like *Ruta*, this remedy is good for bruises to the periosteum (though it is also good for fractures). Typically, the skin is very black and blue around the injury.

BURNS

The most common type of burn is a first-degree burn: reddening of the skin and pain. A second-degree burn creates blistering, along with redness and pain. A third-degree burn has occurred when all the layers of skin are burned through and the skin appears white or charred black. Medical attention is important for any third-degree burn and whenever a first- or second-degree burn extends over a significant portion of the body. Although some people do not think medical attention is necessary for sunburns, extensive sunburns in children call for it.

CALENDULA: This is the first remedy to consider for first-degree burns and for scars from previous burns. It is a good external remedy for sunburns. Apply the diluted tincture, spray, or gel externally.

CANTHARIS: This remedy is for the pain of a burn, especially more severe burns such as second- or third-degree burns. It should be taken either internally in potency or externally or both, though access to the tincture requires a doctor's prescription (this is because the tincture is toxic if taken internally). Internal or external applications of *Cantharis* are good for sunburns.

Causticum: This is an internal remedy for second-degree burns.

BURNS

URTICA URENS: This medicine reduces the pain of first-degree burns, including sunburns, and speeds up the healing process. It can be taken internally in 6th or 30th potency as well as applied in an external tincture.

CANKER SORES

BORAX: This is a primary remedy for canker sores, either in the mouth or on the tongue. It should be taken internally.

CALENDULA: Rinse the mouth with a slightly diluted tincture.

CALCAREA CARB: Use this remedy for newborns who get canker sores.

Mercurius: This is the best remedy for canker sores when the child salivates excessively. (Without excessive salivation, consider *Borax*.)

SULPHURIC ACID: When an infant develops canker sores, this is the first medicine to consider.

CARSICKNESS. See Motion Sickness.

CHICKENPOX

ACONITUM: This remedy should be considered during the initial stages of chickenpox when there is fever, restlessness, and increased thirst.

Antimonium crudum: Most characteristic of these children is their white-coated tongue and their irritable disposition. Other

CHICKENPOX

indications for this remedy are when the child has pimples and pustules that itch, especially after a bath or exposure to water, in the evening, and from the heat of bed. The child tends to feel a prickly heat which is aggravated by exercise and warmth.

Apis: The child has itching and stinging chickenpox that is worse with heat and in warm rooms and better in cold and in cool rooms.

Belladonna: Use *Belladonna* for chickenpox that is accompanied by severe headache, flushed face, hot skin, and drowsiness with the inability to sleep.

RHUS TOX: This is the most common remedy for chickenpox. This child has intense itching, especially at night and from scratching. He is very restless.

~

CIRCUMCISION

ARNICA: This remedy should be given before and after the procedure, to reduce the shock.

STAPHYSAGRIA: This remedy helps to relieve the pain of circumcision. It should be given shortly after circumcision and thirty to sixty minutes after *Arnica*.

~

COLD SORES
(Herpes)

The following homeopathic medicines are often effective in reducing acute herpetic eruptions, though you should seek constitutional treatment from a professional homeopath to prevent future eruptions.

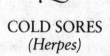

COLD SORES

Mercurius: This is a common remedy for children who have herpes and who drool. A high fever may accompany the symptoms.

NATRUM MUR: The child has lip herpes with extremely dry lips and is very thirsty. He may develop the eruption after an emotional experience. You should try the 6th potency of this remedy first, and if it doesn't work, consider *Rhus tox.*

RHUS TOX: The child has dry and cracked lips and doesn't sleep well.

COLIC

AETHUSA: When this infant is unable to digest milk, it can lead to colic, diarrhea, nausea, or vomiting. The child regurgitates the milk or other food within one hour of eating or drinking, sometimes with violent or projectile vomiting. The vomit usually contains yellow or green curds. The infant sweats and feels very weak, and becomes restless, anxious, and weepy.

Allium cepa: Consider this remedy when an infant has colic along with cold symptoms.

BELLADONNA: The infant has spasms that come and go quickly. She shrieks and involuntarily bends forward or arches backward. Her abdomen will actually feel hot to the touch. She is restless and may also be constipated.

Bryonia: This remedy is for infants who have pain that is aggravated by any motion or pressure. The pain may make them very irritable. The pain is also aggravated by being jarred or being in warm rooms. The baby prefers to lie still with the knees drawn up to relax the abdomen.

COLIC

Calcarea carb: This remedy is primarily effective for the infant who fits the *Calc* type (see "General Characteristics" in part 4). The baby is cold, sweats easily, and has a sour smell and sour discharges. The condition is aggravated by exposure to cold.

CHAMOMILLA: It is commonly given to irritable, colicky infants who are teething at the same time. They have a distended abdomen, and passing gas does not ameliorate the symptoms. The infant doubles up, kicks, and screams. The abdomen is very sensitive to touch. The baby gets some relief from external heat and from being carried and rocked, though this only provides temporary relief. The child may vomit or retch and may also be covered with a cold sweat. The child may also have green, foul-smelling diarrhea containing undigested food.

COLOCYNTHIS: The infant doubles up, and will cry or scream if someone tries to take him out of this position. The baby feels some relief from pressure: either from pushing his own fist into his stomach, leaning against something, or simply lying on his stomach. In the meantime, the baby writhes in pain, and is restless and irritable. The child may have diarrhea at the same time, especially after eating fruit.

Lycopodium: The infant has gas and bloats after anything he eats. The baby doesn't like anything tight around the abdomen because the pressure aggravates him. The worst bloating usually occurs between 4:00 P.M. and 8:00 P.M.; sometimes he wakes with colic at 4:00 A.M. Warm drinks provide some relief, but the symptoms are particularly aggravated by cold drinks, oysters, milk, peas, beans, cabbage, and pastry (either indirectly, because one of these has been eaten by a breast-feeding mother, or directly, eaten by the infant himself). The baby is aggravated by warm rooms and prefers open air.

MAGNESIA PHOS: The infant tends to lie in a fetal position with her knees drawn up. She experiences some relief from

COLIC

warmth, warm applications, hot water, bending double, or eating. Although she has abdominal distention and gas, her pain is not relieved by belching. The bloating will lead the infant to try to loosen her clothing.

NATRUM PHOS: This medicine is one of the generic remedies for colic when there are no distinctive symptoms that suggest another medicine.

Nux vomica: Use for an irritable infant that wants to vomit but can't. The baby also strains to defecate but can't. The symptoms are aggravated after eating. The child is very chilly. Breast-feeding infants may develop their symptoms after their mother eats a rich or spicy meal or if the mother drinks alcohol or takes drugs (either recreational or medicinal).

PULSATILLA: The infant typically develops a distended abdomen in the evening after eating, especially if the infant or breast-feeding mother eats fruit, fats, pastries, or ice cream. The baby may have rumbling and gurgling in the abdomen. Diarrhea may alternate with constipation, and the stools change so often that it seems no stools are alike. The diarrhea may be watery, greenish, and worse at night. The baby may feel relieved by being picked up and rocked.

COMMON COLD

Not every cold needs to be treated, since the body's natural reaction to the cold virus is a healthy response. Consider treating a cold if the symptoms disturb the child badly, if the condition lingers, or if the child needs to attend a special event without suffering respiratory problems.

ACONITUM: This remedy is useful primarily during the first twenty-four hours of a cold. Typically, the child develops her cold or cough after being exposed to dry cold weather. She wakes up with a dry, croupy cough, especially worse at night and after midnight. She has a dry mouth, shortness of breath, and can't spit. The cough is worse from being cold, drinking cold water, from tobacco smoke, lying on either side, and at night.

ALLIUM CEPA: This common remedy for colds is effective when the child has a profuse, watery, burning nasal discharge that is worse in a warm room and better in the open air. The nasal discharge will irritate the child's nostrils, causing pain from simply wiping his nose. He may also have profuse bland (non-burning) tearing from the eyes. He has reddened eyes and a tendency to rub them. He also tends to have a raw feeling in the nose with a tingling sensation as well as violent sneezing. Sometimes the discharge starts in the left nostril and moves to the right. The child may occasionally experience a congestive headache in the front part of his head.

Anas barbariae: Although this medicine (commonly marketed as *Oscillococcinum*) is primarily effective in treating influenza, homeopaths have also found it helpful in treating the common cold. There are no known symptoms from which to individualize treatment, though it is often very effective when used within forty-eight hours of the onset of symptoms. Consider giving it at the first sign of a cold or if you don't know which other medicine to give.

Arsenicum: The child has a burning nasal discharge that irritates the nostrils and upper lip. He is chilly and sensitive to drafts. He may sneeze because of any change in temperature. Typically, the cold begins in the nose and moves down to the throat (once it goes down into the chest a different remedy is usually needed). He also has a dry mouth that makes him very thirsty but for only sips of water at a time.

Belladonna: This remedy should be considered when the nasal discharge suddenly stops and is replaced by a congestive, usually throbbing, headache and high fever.

COMMON COLD

Bryonia: As with the child who needs *Belladonna,* there is little or no nasal discharge but there is a prominent, dull pain over the forehead. The child sneezes often, which may cause a stitching pain on the top of the head. The less the nasal discharge, the more painful becomes the headache. The mouth is dry, as well as the throat, and she may also have a dry cough. She is very thirsty for cold drinks. She feels worse in a warm room.

Calcarea carb: This remedy is for infants or children who experience frequent colds and who fit the typical *Calc carb* syndrome (see "General Characteristics" in part 4). The child is chilly and very sensitive to anything cold, though he prefers to drink ice drinks. He may develop the cold after being chilled. He sweats profusely and it smells sour. So too, the stools. Typically, the child is fair-skinned and pudgy with poor muscle tone. He may get a sore throat at the same time with a swelling of the tonsils and lymph nodes. He has a thick yellowish nasal discharge and rattling respiration due to loose mucus in the throat and chest.

EUPHRASIA: For children who have profuse burning tears from the eyes and bland nasal discharge. The whites of the eyes and the cheeks become reddened from the burning tears. The eye symptoms are worse in the open air. The profuse bland nasal discharge, often accompanied by sneezing, is worse at night, while lying down, and in windy weather. After a day or two of these profuse discharges, the cold then moves to the larnyx, creating a hard cough and a hoarse voice. The cough is worse in the daytime and is ameliorated by lying down.

Ferrum phos: This remedy is effective for children who get head colds with nosebleeds or who have blood in their nasal discharge.

Gelsemium: The child has a watery nasal discharge, sneezing, and a feeling of fullness at the root of the nose. Concurrent

COMMON COLD

with this cold may be fever, body aches, general fatigue, aching in the back part of the head, and sometimes a sore throat.

Hepar sulphur: This remedy is indicated for the child who sneezes from the least exposure to cold air. The nasal discharge is thick and yellow, and her nostrils and the bones of her nose are very sore. The nasal passages are sensitive to cold air. Sometimes the child will have a headache at the same time. Typically, the child is sensitive to touch and is generally irritable.

Kali bic: Stringy, ropy, yellow mucus is characteristic. The child has a thick nasal discharge, and may also experience post-nasal drip with sticky mucus and pain at the root of the nose which feels better when pressure is applied there. The child wants to constantly blow his nose. The discharge, along with the sneezing, is made worse by exposure to cold or in the open air. Sometimes he gets a swollen throat which is relieved by warm liquids. A cough may also occur at the same time.

Natrum mur: This remedy is most often given to children who get recurrent colds and whose symptoms match the certain *Natrum mur* characteristics. The child tends to develop the symptoms after an emotional experience, especially after grief. Death, divorce, unrequited love, or homesickness may cause grief that is not fully expressed, eventually leading to physical complaints. The child sneezes often and has a profuse, watery discharge from the nose and eyes, and loss of taste and smell. Eventually, the nasal discharge may lead to a state of chronic nasal congestion with thick white mucus. The symptoms are worse in the morning, at which time the child usually coughs up mucus. Dry and cracked lips or a cold sore may accompany the cold.

Nux vomica: The child develops his cold after overindulging in food, alcohol, or drugs (medicinal or recreational) or after prolonged mental or emotional stress. The nose alternates

COMMON COLD

between having a watery discharge and being dry and blocked. The discharge is usually flowing steadily in the daytime and obstructed at night. This medicine is also a common remedy for newborns with the sniffles.

PULSATILLA: This remedy is commonly given to the child who gets acute or chronic colds. Typically, there is a thick, yellow or greenish mucus, and a bland discharge (a discharge that does not irritate or burn the nostrils or skin). The nasal congestion is worse at night, especially upon lying down, which leads to mouth-breathing during sleep. The nasal congestion tends to alternate sides of the nose, and is worse in a warm room, flowing more freely in the open air. The child sometimes develops the cold after overindulging in fatty or rich foods. Despite having a dry mouth, the child is not thirsty. *Pulsatilla* is a common remedy for the sniffles in newborns, especially when the nasal discharge is yellow or green. The children who most commonly fit the *Pulsatilla* characteristics are emotional, sensitive, and easily hurt. They are moody and weep easily. They crave affection and sympathy and cannot get enough of it. They are impressionable, so much so that if parents are worried about their child's health, the child will tend to get worse, while if parents are confident that the child will get better, the child usually does.

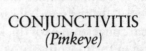

CONJUNCTIVITIS
(Pinkeye)

Apis: The child has itchy and burning eyes and hot tears. The eyelids swell, especially the upper lid, though there may be a bag-like swelling under the eye as well. The eyelid is very sensitive to touch, and it may feel like there is sand in the eye. The child may be hypersensitive to light but cannot bear to have his eyes covered. This remedy is of special value for eye burns caused by bright sunshine on the snow. It is also a common remedy for conjunctivitis in infants.

Arsenicum: Children who need this remedy have bright red, bloodshot eyes. The eyes feel hot and throbbing, tear copiously, and are aggravated by light.

BELLADONNA: The child has pink, even red, eyes. There is burning pain in the eyes, dilated pupils, and hypersensitivity to light.

Calendula: Use this remedy along with an internal remedy. Dilute one part *Calendula* tincture to approximately ten parts water. Use a sterile dropper to place a couple of drops in the eye. This remedy is also often useful after any trauma to the eye.

EUPHRASIA: This remedy is often helpful for conjunctivitis in children who have it as the result of an allergy. The lid margins look and feel sore. There may be pus discharge and constant blinking.

Ferrum phos: This remedy should be considered during the early stages of conjunctivitis when there are few characteristic symptoms.

Hepar sulphur: When the eye and eyelid are very sensitive to touch and to any cold air or cold application, consider this remedy. The child may also have a profuse discharge and be hypersensitive to light.

Mercurius: Rarely given during the onset of conjunctivitis, this remedy is more often helpful for the child who has had pinkeye for at least a couple of days. The child tends to have a profuse burning discharge that is aggravated at night and by heat.

Pulsatilla: The child's eyes burn and itch at night and water profusely in the open air. There may be a thick yellow or white discharge that tends to glue the lids together when the child

CONJUNCTIVITIS

first wakes up in the morning. The eyes are very sensitive to light and are better from cold applications.

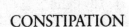

CONSTIPATION

Homeopathic medicines are often effective in treating the acute symptoms of constipation. Increased ingestion of fiber-rich foods is also highly recommended.

Alumina: The child has no urge to have a bowel movement or will tend to have great difficulty, even with small or soft stools. The stools are usually hard, dry, and knotty, and the rectum is sore, dry, and sometimes inflamed. The child may be reacting to eating food cooked in aluminum cookware. He craves dry rice, dry food, and potatoes, yet his constipation is worse from starch, especially potatoes. Not only are the stools sluggish, the child is generally fatigued as well.

BRYONIA: The child has large, hard, dry stools and difficulty expelling them. The tongue is usually coated white. The child is grumpy and wants to be left alone. He is aggravated by any motion and will try to remain as still as possible. He is sensitive to light and prefers to sit in a darkened room. He is aggravated by warm rooms and heat and prefers open air and cool rooms. His mouth and throat are dry; he's very thirsty and craves cold drinks.

CALCAREA CARB: Sometimes a child actually feels better when he is constipated; if so, this remedy should be considered. The child smells sour, and has sour-smelling stools, sweat, and vomit. He is physically lethargic and lacks stamina. He craves eggs—especially soft-boiled—carbohydrates, ice cream, sweets, and salt. He may even crave indigestible items like dirt and chalk. He wants ice drinks (the colder, the better) and is usually averse to hot foods, slimy foods, and mixed foods such as casseroles. He may dislike milk or may be allergic to it. This allergy to milk can lead to constipation, diarrhea, indigestion, or other problems.

NUX VOMICA: The child is constipated with a constant, ineffectual urge to pass stool but with the feeling of never being finished. The onset of constipation sometimes comes after overindulging in food or medical drugs or after prolonged mental or emotional stress. The child feels a need to loosen his pants around the waist. There is concurrent nausea and vomiting, with a sense of relief after vomiting. There may also be heartburn, bloating, gas, or headache.

Sepia: Like children who need *Nux vomica*, children who need *Sepia* have constipation typified by ineffectual urging. When a stool is finally passed, it is sometimes relatively soft, despite the great strain to expel it. The child may also have the sensation of a ball in the rectum. These children develop digestive upsets, constipation, or nasal congestion from milk and milk products.

Silicea: When a child has a *bashful* stool, that is, a stool that is partially expelled but then slips back into the rectum, consider giving *Silicea*. The child has great difficulty passing a stool, even a soft stool. In extreme cases, the child rarely wants to pass a stool at all. She is chilly, averse to cold, but craves cold foods and drinks and is averse to warm foods. She may also crave indigestible items like dirt or chalk.

COUGH

Homeopathic medicines are often effective in treating the acute symptoms of coughs, though professional constitutional care is usually necessary when there are chronic respiratory problems.

COUGH

ACONITUM: The child wakes from sleep with a dry, hoarse, croupy cough, which tends to be worse at night and after midnight. She tends to develop a cold or cough during dry, cold weather. Along with her dry cough, she has a dry mouth and shortness of breath. She is usually very thirsty. The cough is worse from being cold, drinking cold water, from tobacco smoke, lying on either side, and at night, especially after midnight. This remedy is very commonly given for the initial stages of croup, bronchitis, pleurisy, and pneumonia. The child is often restless and anxious.

Antimonium tart: The child has a loud rattling cough with an inability to expectorate mucus. Sometimes coming after being angered or annoyed, the respiratory difficulties cause him to feel drowsy and feeble. The symptoms are usually worse at 4:00 A.M. His difficulty in breathing makes him sit up rather than lie down. Along with these breathing difficulties he is anxious, restless, and irritable. He feels chilly but dislikes stuffy, warm rooms; he wants cool rooms and open windows. This remedy is rarely given at the beginning of an illness.

Belladonna: When cough symptoms appear suddenly and the child has a dry cough with laryngitis, consider this remedy. The children is restless, drowsy, and has wild dreams. The symptoms are worse at night.

BRYONIA: When a common cold starts with a nasal discharge and then moves down into the chest, *Bryonia* is often given, especially when the cough is dry and made worse by motion or by breathing in; the child tends to hold her chest as she breathes in order to limit the motion of the chest and to control the pain. The cough is also aggravated by warm rooms and by eating. She is sensitive to drafts and is always catching cold. She may feel some tickling in the larynx which irritates the cough. Sometimes nausea and vomiting or a headache accompany the cough.

COUGH

Drosera: Bouts of continuous, dry, barking coughing are characteristic of the child who needs this remedy. He feels a spasmodic, tickling cough that is accompanied by choking, cold sweats, and vomiting. The cough is aggravated by lying down and is worse after midnight, especially at 2:00 A.M. The cough is irritated by talking, eating, or drinking cold fluids. He holds onto his chest during the coughing spells because of the pain. He is very chilly and perspires profusely, especially at night. He may also develop a deep, hoarse voice.

Ferrum phos: The child who will benefit from this remedy does not get symptoms that arise suddenly, nor are the symptoms very intense. She may, however, be anemic and become ill after being exposed to cold. The cough becomes worse from cold air, in early morning, and after eating. It is a dry hacking cough, and the expectoration may have some blood in it. She may experience a stitching pain on breathing in and during a cough. She usually has a poor appetite, dislikes meat and milk, preferring sour foods. Hoarseness may accompany the cough.

Hepar sulphur: This remedy is good for a barking, croupy cough, especially when it is worsened by exposure to cold. The cough may also be excited by dryness or dust in the larynx, eating or drinking cold things, breathing deeply, or by a draft. There may be much coughing up of mucus or rattling in the chest without the ability to cough the mucus out. The child sweats during his coughing spells, and may actually feel better in damp weather. He is very irritable while ill.

Ipecac: The child has a hacking cough with a tendency to retch or vomit. There is blood-stained mucus, constriction of the chest, and a tickling in the throat, causing a cough. The child tends to cough with every breath and salivates excessively. The cough is worse in hot, humid weather or in changing weather. She may also sneeze and be hoarse. This remedy is a common medicine for infants with a cough along with vomiting.

COUGH

Kali bic: The child frequently coughs up stringy, ropy, yellow mucus, and is worse after eating, drinking, being uncovered during cold weather, and at 3:00 A.M. He experiences some relief from expectorating the stringy mucus; warmth, warm weather, and lying down in a warm bed also bring relief. He has a sensation of a hair in the back of his throat that irritates the cough. He may have a hoarse voice and feels pain from sticking out his tongue. In some instances he has a pain in the mid-sternum extending through to the back. This remedy is not useful at the beginning stages of a cough.

PHOSPHORUS: The child has a dry hard cough, sometimes with a persistent tickle felt behind the sternum. The cough is aggravated by lying down, especially on the left side, and she wakes up at night, needing to sit up and cough. She is also aggravated by talking, moving, going from a warm room to cold air, or by strong odors. To decrease pain from coughing, she usually holds her chest. The tightness in the chest is relieved by the warmth of a bed. She craves ice drinks. Her illness exhausts her, and she sometimes has an empty, all-gone feeling or a sensation of burning in the chest. The nasal discharge may have some blood streaked in it, and she may become hoarse. This medicine is commonly given for more serious respiratory conditions like pneumonia.

PULSATILLA: This remedy is related to some cough symptoms but is more commonly prescribed based on a child's general characteristics (see part 4). The cough symptoms are aggravated in a warm room or warm weather, by lying down to sleep, and at night. Walking in the cool air provides some relief. Also, the child must sit up in bed to breathe better. Typically, she has a dry cough during the day, and a productive cough with yellow or greenish expectoration at night and upon waking. The key general characteristics of children who will benefit from *Pulsatilla* are that they are affectionate, moody, weepy, indecisive, and always try to please others.

COUGH

They crave affection and sympathy and cannot get enough of it. They have fears of being abandoned, so when parents get ready to go out, for whatever reason, these children may beg them not to leave.

RUMEX: The most distinctive characteristic of children who need this remedy is that their coughs are extremely sensitive to cold air; they may even place blankets or towels over their heads to avoid breathing cold air. They experience ticklings in their throats and irritations below their larynxes that are aggravated by touching or pressing the pits of their throats. They have dry coughs and usually become hoarse. The symptoms are aggravated during the night and also made worse by motion. The child feels better when warm.

SPONGIA: This is one of the primary medicines for a dry, barking, croupy cough. The air passages are dry, sputum is absent, and the child is hoarse. The coughing can be exacerbated by cold air, warm rooms, tobacco smoke, talking, lying with the head low, drinking cold fluids, or eating sweets. The cough also tends to be worse in the early part of the night. Warm foods or drinks, even in small doses, provide some relief, as does sitting up and leaning forward. This remedy is considered a second-stage croup remedy, after *Aconitum* and before *Hepar* and *Kali bic.*

CROUP. See Cough.

CUTS

CALENDULA: This remedy is best suited for clean cuts with little or no infection. Use a tincture (slightly diluted with water), gel, spray, or ointment and apply directly to the wound.

CUTS

Do not use *Calendula* externally on deep cuts because it has such rapid healing capabilities that it will tend to close up a deep cut before it is adequately healed underneath.

HYPERICUM: This remedy is for infected or deep cuts; apply *Hypericum* spray or slightly diluted tincture externally. If there is much shooting or cutting pain, give *Hypericum* 6 or 30 internally.

STAPHYSAGRIA: Give this medicine internally for a deep clean cut or a stab wound.

DIAPER RASH

Chronic diaper rash that is caused by a fungus is best treated by professional medical and homeopathic care.

Calcarea carb: Consider this remedy when diaper rash is chronic. (See "General Characteristics" in part 4.)

CALENDULA: Apply the gel or spray directly on the affected area. *Calendula* can be used concurrently with either internal remedy.

Sulphur: Consider this remedy when diaper rash is chronic. (See "General Characteristics" in part 4.)

DIARRHEA

Chronic or persistent diarrhea can create dehydration and lead to serious health problems. Encourage fluid intake as long as diarrhea continues. Long-lasting or recurrent diarrhea should receive medical supervision, and homeopathic constitutional care should be sought concurrently.

DIARRHEA

AETHUSA: When children are unable to digest milk—leading to colic, diarrhea, nausea, and vomiting—this remedy should be considered. The child regurgitates the milk or other food within an hour of eating, sometimes with violent vomiting. The vomit usually contains yellow or green curds. The infant or child sweats, feels very weak, and becomes restless and weepy.

ARSENICUM: When children have symptoms of food poisoning or stomach flu, this remedy should be the first considered. These children get frequent attacks of offensive-smelling diarrhea. There is usually pain during the diarrhea and discomfort afterward. The child tends to be tired and weak yet also restless, unable to stay in one position for long. Various digestive symptoms accompany the diarrhea, including vomiting, which may start in the middle of the night. The child may feel burning in his abdomen and will have burning stools that irritate the anus. Despite these burning sensations, he is chilly, especially the hands and feet; the symptoms are aggravated by cold. Warmth and warm drinks provide temporary relief. These children are thirsty but only for sips of water at a time.

CALCAREA CARB: This remedy is particularly common for infants, especially during teething. These children usually have sour stools and sour body odor, sweat, and vomit. They have pale stools that lack bile pigment. They crave eggs—especially soft-boiled—carbohydrates, ice cream, sweets, and salt. They may even crave indigestible items like dirt and chalk. They also want ice drinks (the colder, the better). They usually reject hot foods, slimy foods, and mixed foods such as casseroles. They may dislike milk and may be allergic to it, leading to constipation, diarrhea, indigestion, or some other problem. This remedy is often prescribed based on its general characteristics. (See part 4.)

CHAMOMILLA: *Chamomilla* is one of the most common remedies for an infant who has foul-smelling diarrhea and who is

DIARRHEA

highly irritable. The infant tends to have green diarrhea with undigested food, and distension of the abdomen. Passing gas does not ease gas pains, and the abdomen is very sensitive to touch. The infant doubles up, kicks and screams, and may be covered in a cold sweat. Heat gives some relief. *Chamomilla* is commonly given to infants who have diarrhea during teething.

Cinchona: When children experience a painless though debilitating diarrhea, this remedy should be considered. The diarrhea tends to be worse at night and may even be expelled without warning. Typically, the belly is so distended that it may be as tight as a drum. This distension is accompanied by sour and loud belchings which do not provide relief.

Colocynthis: These children have sharp cramping pains with diarrhea shortly after eating or drinking. The pains are relieved by passing gas, passing a stool, or bending over. There is a frequent urge to pass a stool.

IPECAC: Diarrhea with persistent nausea is characteristic of this remedy. Also characteristic is a clean tongue, despite the nausea. The child salivates frequently and has painful urgings to pass a stool.

Iris: The child has a combination of headache with nausea, vomiting, and diarrhea. He also has colic. The diarrhea causes burning irritation at the anus (see Headaches).

MERCURIUS: This is a common remedy for severe diarrhea or food poisoning. The child has burning, watery stools and sometimes slimy, blood-stained stools. Infants may have green stools. Whatever the stool looks like, it will have an offensive odor, and the child will feel pain before, during, or after passing it. There is a frequent or constant urge and a never-get-done feeling. The anus is raw from the burning stools. The symptoms are worse in the evening and at night. A child may feel pinching in the abdomen along with chills. His symptoms make him feel exhausted.

Nux vomica: Diarrhea from rich or spicy foods or from food poisoning typifies this remedy. The child feels better for a short period after passing a stool, but will have diarrhea again immediately after eating and immediately upon waking. She is chilly and irritable.

PODOPHYLLUM: This remedy is effective for profuse, gushing, sometimes frothy diarrhea. The symptoms are worse in the morning (4:00 A.M. to 10:00 A.M.) and during hot summer days. The child has gurgling sounds in the abdomen and bowels and has the diarrhea shortly after eating. She feels weak, has a sweaty head and her skin feels cold. She is restless at night and grinds her teeth. The liver area may be sore and feels better when rubbed or when she lies on her stomach. The child may have an empty, sinking feeling in the abdomen. This is a common remedy for diarrhea in teething infants.

PULSATILLA: This remedy should be considered when treating children generally helped by *Pulsatilla* (see "General Characteristics" in part 4) or when treating children who have diarrhea after eating too much fruit, greasy or rich foods, cold food or drinks, or after exposure to cold. The diarrhea is usually worse at night. In infants the diarrhea is watery and greenish. When children have diarrhea with changeable stools, consider this remedy.

Silicea: Consider this remedy for infants who fit this medicine's general characteristics and who get diarrhea from their mother's milk.

Veratrum album: This is for simple acute (short-term) diarrhea as well as for severe (profuse) diarrhea. These children are usually very fatigued and have watery diarrhea along with

DIARRHEA

vomiting. They shiver, have cold sweats, and may even collapse. Even their bellies feel cold. Despite their chilliness, they have an unquenchable thirst for iced drinks and may want to suck on an ice cube. If a child has an appetite, he will be hungry for cold foods and avoid warm foods. He won't be able to eat fruit, since it tends to cause diarrhea. The diarrhea may be so severe that it exhausts him.

EARACHE

Homeopathic medicines are often effective in treating the acute symptoms of earache. For chronic ear infections, seek professional homeopathic care.

ACONITUM: Consider this remedy at the onset of an earache. The external ear is usually hot and painful. The child feels throbbing pain after exposure to cold, and he is hypersensitive to noise or music. A fever generally accompanies the ear infection, and the child may also have a dry cough and a congested nose. He tends to be very thirsty.

Allium cepa: This remedy is helpful when children have a cold with their ear infection. Their cold includes a burning, watery, nasal discharge that irritates the nostrils. They also may have sore throats with pains that extends to the ears. Their symptoms are worse in a warm room and better in cool and open air.

BELLADONNA: This is a commonly prescribed remedy for ear infection when the child has a reddened ear, ear canal, or eardrum, and sometimes a flushed face. The symptoms come on suddenly, sometimes after getting a haircut or exposure to a cold draft. Usually the right ear is affected more than the left. The pains are throbbing, piercing, and sometimes extend to the throat; motion aggravates them and they are worse at night. The child feels better sitting semi-erect and is soothed by warm applications. The ears sting, inside and out. The child may have a fever at the same time—usually a high fever—with a sore throat that feels hot. The child may also have swollen glands. Emotionally, the child is agitated and in extreme cases may become delirious and will bite and scream. *Belladonna* is not commonly used if the child has had an earache for more than three days.

Calcarea carb: This remedy is more often prescribed based on the child's general characteristics than on his specific ear symptoms. These children are chilly, very sensitive to anything cold (though they prefer to drink ice drinks) and may develop their ear infection after being chilled. Despite being chilly, the child's head is hot, and it sweats profusely. His sweat and stools smell sour. Typically, the child is fair-skinned and pudgy with poor muscle tone. He may get a sore throat at the same time with swelling on the tonsils and lymph glands. He also tends to be constipated. The ear pain is usually throbbing; the ear discharge is thick, yellow, offensive-smelling and is aggravated by cold wind.

CHAMOMILLA: Children who need this common remedy for ear infection are in great pain and are extremely irritable because of it. They demand things but refuse them once they are offered. They are impatient and cannot be consoled. They are very sensitive to touch, though they feel temporary relief by being rocked or carried. The pains are aggravated by exposure to cold air, especially cold winds. The ear infection sometimes results from being exposed to cold. The tearing pains in the ears lead them to cry—usually loudly. The ears feel stuffed up, and there may be buzzing in them. Infants may be teething at the same time that they have this kind of ear infection.

Ferrum phos: Like *Aconitum* and *Belladonna*, this remedy is given during the first stages of inflammation. But unlike these

EARACHE

other remedies, the symptoms of the child who needs *Ferrum phos* have a slower onset and are less intense. The earache is usually on the left side.

Hepar sulphur: This remedy is often used when there are no other distinguishing symptoms except the child being physically and psychologically hypersensitive. The ears are extremely sensitive to touch and cold and may be relieved by heat and by warm applications. The child is irritable and throws tantrums. He usually feels sharp, sometimes splinter-like pains in the ear, and the ear discharge smells offensive. The child may have a dry, perhaps croupy, cough along with his earache.

Lycopodium: These children have ear infections that are either worse on the right side or that start on the right and move to the left. The pains are worse between 4:00 P.M. and 8:00 P.M., or when the child is exposed to cold air, drafts, or when he lies on the right side. His ear feels stopped-up and sometime he hears ringing and buzzing. The ear discharge is usually thick, yellow, and burning. Typically, children who need *Lycopodium* tend to have digestive symptoms, including gas and bloating, either prior to or during ear infections. The child is usually anxious and insecure, and always wants someone around—at least in a nearby room. He constantly worries about what others think of him and is afraid to try anything new. He may be quite boastful, and may even be a bully (as a way to hide his deep insecurities).

MERCURIUS: This remedy is the most common remedy for children with chronic ear infections, though it is also used for certain acute problems. There is pus and a gluey, burning, and offensive-smelling discharge that is green or sometimes yellow (a concurrent cold or eye infection may also have a greenish discharge). The pain and discharge are both worse at night and from the warmth of bed. There may be ringing or pulsations in the ear, and the ear pain tends to extend from the

EARACHE

throat to the ear. The child may also have a sore throat with swollen glands and bad breath. There may be various kinds of ear pain: burning, bursting, pinching, pressing, or shooting pain that will be aggravated by hot or cold applications, the warmth of bed, or by stooping, and will be relieved by blowing the nose. These children tend to have a stopped sensation in their ears and may also have eruptions behind their ears. They may drool a great deal, soaking their pillows, and sweat so much that their sheets get wet. Two different types of *Mercurius* are useful if the above description fits but the child's earache is one-sided: use *Mercurius iodatus flavus* if right-sided or *Mercurius iodatus ruber* if left-sided.

Plantago: When children have a earache with teething or tooth pain, this remedy should be considered. The child may also have pain that goes from one ear through the head to the other ear. This remedy is most effective in its tincture—diluted slightly in water—placing a couple of drops directly in the ear. To alleviate the tooth pain, rub the tincture directly on the gums.

MULLEIN: This remedy is most effective when a couple of drops of oil (called *Mullein* oil) are placed directly in the ear. It is best for the child who feels pain with a sense of the ear being blocked-up. The ear canal is dry and scaly. *Mullein* should not be given if there is any ear discharge. Because it is applied externally, it can be given along with any of the other remedies that are taken internally.

PULSATILLA: This common remedy for ear infections may be prescribed when the earache starts after the child has gotten wet or been chilled. The ear problem often comes with or after a cold. The ear pains are worse at night and when the child is warm in bed; some relief is felt from cool applications. Usually there is little pain during the day. If there is a discharge, it is thick, bland, yellow or greenish. The child may feel his ear is

EARACHE

stopped. A sore throat, cough, or fever may be concurrent. Although he may not be thirsty, he prefers cold drinks and refuses warm drinks. These children are gentle, mild, and weepy. Although their pain will make them somewhat irritable, it is more whining than anger. Likewise, their crying will be sweet and quiet, the kind that makes you want to hug them. Since these children love sympathy and affection, they are soothed by this attention. They also feel better when you rock them.

EYE INJURIES

Except for minor blows to the face which create a simple black eye, eye injuries need prompt medical attention. The following medicines should be given to the child on the way to the doctor's office.

ACONITUM: Called the *Arnica* of the eye, this remedy is the first to consider for injuries to the eye (also when the child is extremely restless and fearful after an eye injury). It is also effective for a black eye with minor trauma to the eyeball itself. It's also a good choice when a child gets dust, sand, or a foreign object in the eye, and then—in his efforts to wipe his eyes—he accidentally cuts his cornea. *Aconitum* helps to relieve the pain and to heal these injuries. It is primarily indicated as soon after the injury as possible.

ARNICA: This remedy is the best for the shock of the injury and to help the body absorb the blood under the skin. External application of *Arnica* ointment, gel, or spray should be used only if the skin has not been broken. Do not put any *Arnica* preparation in the eye. Internal and external applications can be taken at the same time.

CALENDULA: *Calendula* tincture can be used concurrently with any of the other remedies when they are being taken internally. For mild scratches on the cornea, dilute *Calendula* tincture with sterilized water (one part tincture and ten parts water) and drop into the affected eye.

LEDUM: This is the primary remedy for a black eye. It is effective in treating pain along with the black and blue discoloration, especially when the child feels relief when cold is applied.

SYMPHYTUM: This remedy should be considered for injuries to the eyeball or cheekbone from a blow to the face. It should also be considered to heal older injuries to the tissue around the eye or to the eyeball itself, or when *Aconitum* has not worked fast enough.

FEVER

Children with fevers higher than 103.5 degrees (taken orally) that do not respond to the above remedies or general home care within six hours need professional medical care. Infants less than six months old should receive medical care for any fever higher than 100.5 degrees. Infants less than two months old should receive medical care for any fever. Also, when a child has any fever with extreme irritability, lethargy, and mental confusion along with stiffness of the neck, seizures, recurrent vomiting, or labored breathing, seek medical care immediately.

ACONITUM: This should be considered only at the beginning stages of a fever. The fever comes on suddenly, usually after the child has been chilled. She has chills with her fever and is easily chilled when uncovered. She may have a red face or alternate between being pale and being red. She is thirsty.

FEVER

ARSENICUM: The child has a fever and is very thirsty, but only for sips of water at a time. He tends to have his highest temperature between midnight and 3:00 A.M. He is restless and anxious. He is very chilly and feels better when warmed.

BELLADONNA: When children have a sudden onset of high fever with flushed faces and reddened lips, this remedy is the first to consider. These children also tend to have hot heads and cold extremities. The skin is usually so hot that it radiates heat (you can feel it by placing your hand a couple of inches away from the skin). The fever is a dry heat, without perspiration. The child tends to have a strong and bounding pulse. At night the temperature gets its highest, making the child agitated, sometimes delirious, perhaps leading her to hallucinate.

FERRUM PHOS: Like *Aconitum* and *Belladonna,* this remedy is given at the first stages of fever. Unlike with these other remedies, the child who needs *Ferrum phos* has a slower onset of fever and less intensity of symptoms.

Nux vomica: This remedy should be considered when the child has a fever as a side effect of a drug, after overeating, or from loss of sleep. Chilliness may accompany the fever, with a worsening of symptoms when the child is uncovered. There may also be, at the same time, head pain or digestive symptoms such as constipation, diarrhea, or indigestion.

Pulsatilla: These children have fevers with chills and are worse in warm rooms. They want open air but need to be properly covered. They are not thirsty.

Sulphur: Like *Belladonna,* the child has a fever with red skin. A characteristic symptom is that she has diarrhea that drives her out of bed in the early morning. She is also very thirsty and sweats profusely; the sweat has an offensive smell.

FEVER

FLU
See Influenza.

FOOD POISONING
See also Diarrhea and Indigestion.

Food poisoning can lead to severe vomiting or diarrhea. These symptoms are usually short-lived, but if they persist, seek professional medical care.

ARSENIUM: This is the most common remedy for food poisoning. The child has frequent bouts of offensive-smelling and burning diarrhea, which rapidly creates an irritation of the anus. The child also feels nauseous and will usually have burning vomit that irritates the throat. She is chilly and feels worse when exposed to the cold. The worst symptoms occur at or after midnight. The child is restless and constantly changes position, especially in bed, and she may get sick enough to feel very weak. Her abdomen is sensitive to touch, though it feels better when warmth is applied. Warm drinks may also be soothing. There are burning pains in the stomach that are worse from most foods or drinks (especially cold foods or drinks, which are quickly vomited), from taking a deep breath, or from the slightest touch. She is thirsty but takes only sips of water at a time.

Mercurius: These children have burning, watery stools and sometimes slimy, blood-stained stools. Infants may have green stools. Whatever the stools look like, they smell bad, and the children will feel pain before, during, or after passing them. They have constant urges to do so but never feel done. The anus aches. The symptoms are worse in the evening and at night. The child may feel pinching in the abdomen along with chills. He feels nauseous but vomiting gives no relief. The symptoms exhaust him.

FOOD POISONING

Nux vomica: The diarrhea is caused by rich or spicy foods or by food poisoning. The child feels better briefly after passing a stool, but has diarrhea again immediately after eating or upon waking. She is bloated and has gas along with nausea. She feels better after vomiting. She is chilly and irritable.

FRACTURE
See Bone Injuries.

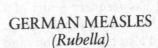

GERMAN MEASLES
(Rubella)

Children with German measles should stay at home until they are well, both for their own health and because of the serious consequences of infecting a pregnant woman with this virus.

Aconitum: This remedy is for the sudden onset of a rash with a fever. The child is usually very thirsty. *Aconitum* is only appropriate during the initial stages of this illness.

Belladonna: When a child experiences a sudden onset of high fever with a flushed face and reddened lips, this remedy is the first to consider. The child tends to have a hot head and cold extremities. The skin is usually so hot that it radiates heat (you can feel it by placing your hand a couple of inches away from the skin). The fever is a dry heat, without perspiration. The child tends to have a strong, bounding pulse. At night the temperature gets its highest, making the child agitated, sometimes delirious, perhaps making him hallucinate when his eyes are closed.

Pulsatilla: The child has chill with her fever. She feels worse in warm rooms. She wants fresh air but needs to be properly covered. She has no thirst and has a flushed face.

GERMAN MEASLES

GRIEF

Homeopathic medicines are often effective in treating the acute symptoms of grief, though professional constitutional care is usually necessary to achieve a deeper level of cure when depression is a chronic condition. Professional psychological care is also suggested when grief is deep or prolonged.

IGNATIA: *Ignatia* is the primary remedy for children who are suffering from grief, especially if they try to hold it in. Usually these children are not successful at suppressing their emotion, and they tend to become hysterical (see "General Characteristics" in part 4).

NATRUM MUR: These children tend to have long-term emotional memories. Once they are emotionally hurt, they do not let go of pain easily; they bear grudges, are resentful, and dwell on past problems. Death, divorce, lack of parental love, or homesickness may cause griefs that are unexpressed, eventually leading to physical complaints. They rarely cry in public. Instead, they retreat to their room and sob when alone. They reject sympathy and want to be left alone.

PULSATILLA: This child is emotional and sensitive. He is easily hurt, weepy, easily discouraged, and easily affected by people and the environment he is in. He can cry for almost any reason but especially if he is criticized and punished or even if he is simply ignored. He never sobs; his tears have a sweetness in them that make you want to hug him. He is also moody, weeping one moment and laughing the next, and prone to self-pity, saying to himself, "Why does this always happen to me?" Once he gets the special attention he wants and needs, his pain disappears and is quickly forgotten. He cannot get enough affection; he soaks it up like a sponge.

Staphysagria: *Staphysagria* is a primary remedy for the child who suppresses her grief and tries to control her feelings: she silently stews about her problems. Her physical ailments begin shortly after this suppression of grief. She can, however, repress her feelings for only so long: eventually, she explodes in rage. She trembles, loses her voice, throws things, demands something but then refuses it once it is offered, has great difficulty concentrating, becomes exhausted, and suffers from insomnia. She is sensitive to the least offense: every word said to her is taken the wrong way. When she finally explodes, she tends to feel bad about it afterward. *Staphysagria* is also a common remedy for children who have been abused, either physically or sexually.

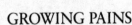

GROWING PAINS

Parents can assume that their child is having growing pains when, during a growth spurt and despite no obvious injury, the child experiences pains in the legs.

CALCAREA PHOS: Used for children whose pain seems to be caused solely by very rapid growth.

Causticum: This remedy should be considered for growing pains that are accompanied by stiffness in or around the joints.

HAY FEVER
See Allergies.

HEADACHES

Homeopathic medicines are often effective in treating the acute symptoms of headache, though professional constitutional care is usually necessary to achieve a deeper level of cure of chronic headaches. Persistent or severe headaches demand a visit to a physician.

HEADACHES

Arsenicum: Children who will benefit from this remedy tend to experience the worst symptoms of their headaches after midnight or from excitement or exertion. They feel better lying down in a dark room, or lying with their heads raised. They experience burning pains, even though they are physically chilly. The head feels better from washing it in cold water or from cold applications. Head pains alternate with other physical symptoms, such as diarrhea. The pains are aggravated by light and motion. The child is restless; he tosses and turns, trying to find a comfortable position. Another type of headache is of a neuralgic nature, with extreme sensitivity of the scalp (combing or brushing the hair may hurt). This latter type of headache is aggravated by cold and relieved by warmth.

BELLADONNA: This remedy is effective for a child whose head feels full, as if it could burst. The pain usually is in the forehead or around the eyes; throbbing pain that is worse by jarring, touching, bending forward, lying flat, or motion of the eyes, and is relieved by gradually applied pressure, sitting up, or bending the head backward. The eyes are sensitive to light and the face is flushed. The child feels dizzy, which becomes worse when stooping.

BRYONIA: Like children who need *Belladonna,* the child who will benefit from *Bryonia* feels as if his head might burst. He feels sharp pain from the slightest motion, even from motion of the eyes, motion of the chest from coughing, or motion of the throat from talking. He must keep perfectly quiet. There is some relief from firm pressure. The pains can come on suddenly, usually upon waking in the morning, and get worse as the day progresses. Usually the child has a throbbing pain in the forehead and behind the eyes. The symptoms are worse in a warm room and from heat, including the heat of the sun. They are also worse from stooping and from strong light. The child wants to sit in the dark. His headache is often the forerunner to other symptoms: respiratory (oppressive heaviness

HEADACHES

in the chest), digestive (constipation is very common), and fever. He is irritable, averse to sympathy and to talking, and prefers being alone.

Calcarea carb: This remedy is more often prescribed based on its general characteristics than on the specific headache symptoms. These children are chilly, very sensitive to anything cold (though they prefer to drink ice drinks), and may develop their headaches after being chilled. Despite being chilly, especially their hands and feet, their heads are hot, and they tend to sweat profusely. Their perspiration and their stools are sour-smelling. Typically, these children are fair-skinned and pudgy with poor muscle tone. They may concurrently get sore throats with swelling on the tonsils and lymph glands. They also tend to be constipated. Their headaches tend to include tearing or splitting pains, which are aggravated by daylight and mental exertion and relieved by lying down in a dark room and by warmth or warm applications. They tend to be dizzy and nauseous as well.

Euphrasia: This child usually has headaches with eye and nose symptoms at the same time. She has stitching pains in the eyes that cut through the head; she feels that her head is going to burst. She may also feel a dull headache in the forehead and a bruised feeling which is worse in the evening. She is sensitive to light. She has burning tears, and a bland runny nose.

GELSEMIUM: Children with headaches who need this remedy feel weak and tired, and seem to be able to open their eyes only halfway. The headache is felt in the back part of the head. The head feels very heavy, as if there were a band around it. The child feels dizzy and may have a staggered gait. He feels worse in the morning, from exposure to sun, from warmth, and from hot, local applications, and feels better after lying down with the head raised by pillows. He also feels relief after profuse

HEADACHES

urination. These children may develop their headaches when they have influenza.

Hepar sulphur: The distinguishing symptom of children with headaches who need this remedy is that their scalps are so sensitive that simply combing their hair may be painful. The child feels like a nail has been thrust into her head. There is boring or bursting pain, especially above the nose. The pains are worse from shaking the head, motion, riding in a car, stooping, moving her eyes, or even from the weight of a hat—though the pains are partially relieved by the firm pressure of a tight bandage wound around the head. The pains also tend to be aggravated by dry weather.

Hypericum: This remedy should be considered when a child develops a headache after a blow to the head or a fall that hurts his spine.

Ignatia: This medicine is useful when children develop headaches after an emotional experience, especially after grief or anxiety. There is a pressing pain as though a nail or blunt instrument were being driven into the skull. The pains are aggravated by talking, tobacco smoke, or strong odors, and are ameliorated by stooping forward, by lying on the same side as the pain, or after passing a large quantity of urine. If the head feels hot, the child feels relief from warm applications.

Ipecac: The child who gets persistent nausea along with his headache often needs this medicine. He tends to have head pain on one side or a bruised, crushed feeling in the head.

Iris: The child has a combination of headache, nausea, vomiting, and diarrhea or constipation. The headache is usually in the front part of the head, often on the right side, with sense of fullness and throbbing, sometimes severe enough to cause dimmed vision. This problem is worse in the spring or autumn, or from 2:00 A.M. to 3:00 A.M., and is aggravated by rest and partially relieved by gentle motion.

HEADACHES

Kali bic: The distinguishing symptoms that accompany the headache are thick, stringy nasal discharge and sinus congestion. The child feels extreme pain at the root of the nose, which feels better when pressure is applied. The bones and scalp feel sore, and there is pain over the eyebrows. The child may develop a migraine with nausea and vomiting, all of which tend to be aggravated when she stands up. The severe pain may lead to dimmed vision. The pains are made worse by cold, light, noise, walking, stooping, and are also worse in the morning (especially on waking or at 9:00 A.M.) or at night. She prefers to lie down in a darkened room, and feels some relief from warmth, warm drinks, or after eating.

Lachesis: The headache is worse on the left side, or it begins on the left side and then moves to the right. The pains are much worse when the child first wakes up in the morning. The head pains are usually felt over the left eye and into the root of the nose. The head is very sensitive to touch: the pressure of a pillow or even a comb in the hair may irritate it. The heat of the sun is also aggravating, although being in the open air provides some relief.

Natrum mur: A throbbing or bursting migraine headache, usually in the front part of the head or on one side or another, is characteristic of children who need this remedy. The child may look pale and feel nauseous. The worst symptoms are between morning and noon. There is some relief while lying down, from vomiting, or after sleep. Another type of headache that *Natrum mur* effectively treats is that of anemic children who tend to be nervous and emotional.

NUX VOMICA: The child has a headache along with nausea and a loathing of food. The symptoms are worse in the morning and from any exertion. They begin while the child is in bed and persist in the open air. The pain is aggravated by stooping, light, noise, exposure to the sun, moving or opening the eyes, or from coughing. Some relief occurs from warmth, quiet, or pressure on the head. There is heaviness of the head and congestive pain. The child sometimes gets migraine headaches. He also often gets constipated.

Phosphorus: Hunger typically precedes or accompanies a headache in a child who needs *Phosphorus,* though the head pain may also result from eating too much sugar. These children are generally chilly and feel worse from cold, though coldness actually relieves their head pains, while warmth aggravates them. There is a heaviness of the head, with burning or pressing pains which are aggravated by warm rooms, by motion, coughing, and by lying down, especially on the right side. The symptoms tend to be worse on the left side, especially over the left eye. The child may experience visual symptoms concurrent with the headache, including photophobia, flickers, or black and white floating spots. Cool air brings relief; cold applications, sleep, wrapping the head up, or eating also help. The skin over the forehead feels very tight. The child may have burning eyes and feel dizzy from rising too rapidly.

Pulsatilla: Children who need this medicine sometimes get their headaches from overeating (especially fats or ice cream), from getting wet, or because of grief. The head pains are worse in the evening, in warm rooms, in bed, when stooping, while blowing the nose, when coughing, after being overheated, from being in the sun too long, after rising from lying down, and after eating. Slow walking helps, as well as being in the open air, cold applications, and lying with the head high. Commonly, these children develop their headaches while at school. When there are head pains in the front of the head, they are often accompanied by digestive problems.

Sanguinaria: Headaches—including migraines—on the right side of the head or over the right eye call for the use of this medicine. Sometimes the head pains start on the right and

HEADACHES

move to the left. The child feels his head is going to burst. The headache usually starts in the morning, increases in intensity until noon, eases up by 3:00 P.M., and significantly decreases in the evening and night. These children become hypersensitive during their headaches and are aggravated by the slightest jar or jolt, as well as by noise, light, and odors. They prefer to lie down in a dark room. There may be nausea and vomiting. There may also be dizziness, especially in the morning, on rising from sitting, or from turning the head quickly. The child tends to lose his appetite and may even develop a disgust for food, but has an insatiable hunger for acidic or spicy things.

Spigelia: Headaches on the left side are characteristic of children who need this medicine. The pains are worse in the daytime and in the sun and better at night. The pains are also worse from any motion (even moving the eyes), from noise, being jarred, or exposure to tobacco smoke, and are often described as stitching or shooting. The pain may be felt in the left eye and extend through to the back of the head. The eyes may feel too large. The head pains may be slightly relieved when the child applies pressure to the head or lies down with the head high.

HEAD INJURIES

Children with a head injury should receive immediate medical care if there is any diminished alertness, slurred speech, memory loss, change of personality, a seizure or convulsion, severe or persistent vomiting, blurred or double vision, pupils of unequal size, severe or persistent headache, difficulty moving the extremities, a clear or bloody fluid coming from the ear or nostril, or a slow, irregular, or weak pulse.

<u>ARNICA:</u> This is the first medicine to give after an injury to the head, whether there is a concussion or not.

HEAD INJURIES

Hypericum: Use this medicine for injuries to the head with shooting pains that extend from the area of injury.

NATRUM SULPH: This medicine should be given if the swelling from a head injury is gone but the pain persists, or when children develop persistent, chronic symptoms, such as headaches, nerve pains, or fatigue. A child who becomes noticeably more depressed or irritable after a head injury will benefit from this medicine. It is also helpful for an infant who experiences a difficult birth, during which trauma to the head may have occurred.

HEATSTROKE

Heatstroke is a medical emergency. The following medicines can be given on the way to the doctor. It is recommended to keep the child cool and, if possible, apply ice packs or a cold sponge to the child's skin.

BELLADONNA: The child has a fever, a throbbing headache, flushed face, and seems to be in a stupor. The head pain is partially relieved by bending the head backward, keeping the head covered, and by sitting quietly.

GLONOINE: This medicine should be considered when the child who has been overexposed to the sun has a fever with waves of heat, throbbing headache, reddened face, and is in a stupor. The head pain is worsened by bending the head backward and by applying cold water, which may cause spasms. The child may feel some relief by uncovering his head or body and by being in the open air.

HEAT EXHAUSTION

The child should be kept cool by applying cold, wet cloths to the skin. He should be given water with a half-teaspoon of salt

HEAT EXHAUSTION

added per glass. If there is loss of consciousness or if symptoms do not improve within an hour, medical care should be sought.

CUPRUM MET: The child feels extremely cold, is pale and covered with clammy sweat, feels weak, faint, and generally stiff all over.

VERATRUM ALBUM: This remedy should be given if the child is chilly with cold and clammy skin, copious cold sweat, and profuse diarrhea that exhausts him.

~

HEPATITIS

It is recommended that infants or children with jaundice or hepatitis get medical supervision because of the occasional complications that they may experience. Homeopathy has much to offer in the treatment of hepatitis.

<u>Aconitum</u>: This remedy is for the initial stages of hepatitis. There is jaundice (yellowing of the skin, tongue, and whites of the eyes) and tenderness in the liver region, high fever, and restlessness. It is especially useful in newborns.

<u>Belladonna</u>: These children have jaundice and intermittent liver pains. The pains are aggravated by breathing, jarring, motion, and lying on the right side.

CHELIDONIUM: The distinguishing symptom of the child who needs this medicine is that she feels pain in the liver region which extends towards the back and shoulder and to the right scapula. She may feel various pains on the right side of her body. The pains are aggravated by motion, touch, and pressure, and are better by heat, warm food, hot drinks, and lying on her left side. She feels a general lethargy and doesn't want to do anything.

LYCOPODIUM: This is one of the primary remedies for hepatitis in children. The child feels a sense of tension like a cord or hoop in the liver area, and he may have difficulty standing upright. He dislikes warm rooms and prefers open air. His lowest energy is between 4:00 P.M. and 8:00 P.M.

Mercurius: In addition to jaundice, the child has a yellow tongue which is swollen and puffy; the teeth leave their impression upon it. He salivates excessively. The liver is swollen and tender, and he has an overall sensitivity to both extremes of temperatures.

Nux vomica: This remedy should be considered in jaundice of infants whose mothers have abused recreational or therapeutic drugs.

PHOSPHORUS: The child has burning pains under the upper right rib cage and between her shoulder blades. The pains are relieved by cold food and ice drinks and are aggravated by warm food and drinks or by touch or pressure. Sometimes the child may vomit after the cold food or drinks have become warmed in her stomach. This medicine is often appropriate for jaundice in newborns.

HIVES

Homeopathic medicines usually act rapidly to reduce the pain and discomfort of this allergic condition. Professional homeopathic care is recommended to cure chronically recurring hives.

APIS: These children experience hives with swelling that is made worse by warmth of any kind. There is puffiness around the face and under the eyes, and swollen eyelids. There is intolerable itching, especially at night in bed. The child's skin feels full, tense, and tight and is hypersensitive.

HIVES

Nux vomica: Children who experience hives concurrent with digestive problems may need this remedy. In addition to sensations of burning and itching, the child has a sensation of numbness in any place that is touched. His symptoms are worse in the early morning or evening and when uncovered.

PULSATILLA: When children develop hives after eating rich or greasy foods or after an emotional experience, this medicine should be considered. Sometimes these children have diarrhea concurrent with their hives.

Rhus tox: Children who get hives shortly after getting wet or chilled should be given this remedy.

Sulphur: Like the child who needs *Apis,* children who need this medicine are hot and itchy, aggravated by warmth of any kind and relieved by coolness. The child also get hives from overexertion or after eating foods to which he is allergic. Typically, his lips become reddened.

URTICA URENS: The hives itch and burn, as though there was a prickly heat on the skin or the skin was scorched. The symptoms are worse when exposed to heat. The child has a constant desire to touch or rub the eruptions. The condition tends to dissipate when the child lays down and rests, but reappears upon rising.

IMPETIGO

Although generally self-limiting, impetigo can spread out of control. If the homeopathic medicine does not reduce the spread of impetigo within forty-eight hours, or if it spreads to a mucous membrane, medical care should be sought.

ANTIMONIUM CRUDUM: This is one of the most commonly given remedies for impetigo. The child has pimples and pus-

IMPETIGO

tules which itch, especially after a bath or exposure to water, or also in the evening and from the heat of bed. She may feel a prickly heat which is aggravated by exercise and warmth. Characteristically, the child has a thickly coated white tongue.

ARSENICUM: The child has impetigo with burning or itching eruptions which are aggravated by scratching, causing additional burning.

Graphites: The distinguishing characteristic is skin eruptions that exude a thick, sticky, honey-colored fluid. The skin around the joints is the most frequently affected. The itching can be severe and is usually worse at night, from heat, and after exposure to water, and is relieved by cold.

Hepar sulphur: The eruptions are sensitive to touch, and there is a tendency for them to ulcerate. There is also a tendency for the child's hands to be cracked and dry; she may also have cracks behind the ears.

PULSATILLA: Children with impetigo who are *Pulsatilla* types (gentle, mild, aggravated by heat, and thirstless) may benefit from this medicine.

Rhus tox: Children with moist eruptions that itch worse at night while in bed will benefit from this remedy.

SULPHUR: There is usually a pre-existing skin condition which the child has aggravated by intense scratching. Though scratching provides some relief, heavy scratching can cause bleeding and may lead to infections like impetigo. The itching is made worse by warmth, especially the warmth of bed. The itching is initially relieved by warm bathing, but fifteen minutes after getting out of the bath the itching is worse than before. There are dry, thick, yellow scabs with a discharge which may irritate the surrounding skin.

IMPETIGO

INDIGESTION
See also Constipation, Diarrhea, or Food Poisoning.

Digestive problems in infants and children could be routine or could be potentially dangerous. Medical supervision should be considered at the same time as homeopathic constitutional care if symptoms persist.

ACONITUM: Digestive problems that occur during very hot weather, especially after drinking ice drinks, may benefit from this remedy. The abdomen is sensitive to touch. These children experience nausea, vomiting, and diarrhea.

Aethusa: When the child is unable to digest milk, leading to colic, diarrhea, nausea, and vomiting, this is a medicine to consider giving. The child regurgitates the milk or other food within one hour of eating or drinking, sometimes with violent or projectile vomiting containing yellow or green curds. The child is cold and clammy, feels very weak, and falls asleep after vomiting. He is also restless, anxious, and weepy.

Antimonium crudum: The child regurgitates milk shortly after drinking it. She is disgusted by all food, although she tends to be thirsty in the evening. She may have watery diarrhea with undigested food particles, which is aggravated by becoming overheated or by eating vinegar or acidic foods. The nausea is particularly common at night and in the early morning. Characteristically, the child has a thickly coated white tongue.

Antimonium tart: There is constant nausea which may be felt in the chest, as well as copious amounts of saliva, and a tongue that is coated white. The child may crave apples and acid drinks but is made worse by them. This medicine is rarely given at the beginning of an illness.

Argentum nit: The child has a strong craving for sweets, even though they tend to cause him problems, especially flatulence.

INDIGESTION

An infant tends to develop diarrhea when their breast-feeding mother eats a lot of sweets. The symptoms are aggravated by warmth in any form and are better with cold, open air.

ARSENICUM: This medicine is as often given based on the child's general characteristics as it is on the nausea and vomiting symptoms. It is one of the most commonly prescribed medicines for diarrhea, though it is also often given for nausea and vomiting. The child is chilly and feels worse if exposed to the cold. She has her worst symptoms at or after midnight. She is restless and constantly changes position, especially in bed, and may get sick enough to feel weak. The abdomen is sensitive to touch, though it feels better from warm applications. Warm drinks also may be soothing. There are burning pains in the stomach that are worse from most foods or drinks (especially cold foods or drinks, which are quickly vomited), taking a deep breath, or the least touch. The child may also have a burning vomit which will irritate the throat and a burning diarrhea which will irritate the anus. She is thirsty but takes only sips of water at a time.

BRYONIA: The child suffers from indigestion after eating rich or fatty foods. The food lies in the stomach undigested and feels like a heavy lump. He feels nauseated and may vomit, usually feeling worst in the morning upon rising. He is aggravated by motion, whether it is rising from the bed, walking, or simply taking a deep breath. He has burning and cutting pains in the stomach or liver. He cannot bear a light touch on the abdomen but can feel relieved by firm pressure. The child is sometimes constipated, has a white-coated tongue, and a headache in the front part of the head.

Calcarea carb: This medicine is as often given based on the general characteristics as it is on the nausea and vomiting symptoms. These children are chilly and very sensitive to anything cold, though they prefer to drink ice drinks. Despite being chilly, the child's head is hot, and it sweats profusely.

INDIGESTION

The perspiration and stools are sour-smelling. Typically, the child is fair-skinned and pudgy with poor muscle tone. He may also get a sore throat with swelling on the tonsils and lymph glands. He has a distended abdomen and tends to be constipated. The vomit, too, is sour-smelling; it is often in curds shortly after nursing or eating. The child suffers indigestion after eating fat or drinking milk.

CHAMOMILLA: Although these children have characteristic physical symptoms, their psychological symptoms tend to be more prominent. Consider this medicine first if a child suffers from digestive problems either before, during, or after a temper tantrum. She is extremely irritable and cross. She demands something but then refuses it once it is offered. Nothing satisfies the child, except being rocked or carried or warm applications on her abdomen—and these only provide temporary relief. The child has a distended abdomen, and passing gas does not ameliorate her symptoms. The child doubles up, kicks, and screams. The abdomen is very sensitive to touch. She may also be covered in a cold sweat. She tends to have green, foul-smelling stools or diarrhea containing undigested food. If she vomits, there is much retching. She doesn't want warm drinks.

Colocynthis: Like *Chamomilla,* this remedy is for children with digestive problems before, during, or after temper tantrums. These children tend to have various types of cramping pains: cutting and gripping cramps in the abdomen which are made worse by eating or drinking, even small amounts; cramps with nausea, diarrhea, and much gas which may be relieved by bending over or when lying on the abdomen. The child may want to hang over a chair or bed in a way which applies pressure to the abdomen. This firm pressure may provide some relief at first, but later the abdomen will be sensitive and aggravated by any touch. Temporary relief can be obtained by warm application, walking, or passing gas or a stool. The child has a bitter taste in his mouth, and his tongue feels burnt or scalded.

INDIGESTION

Ignatia: This medicine should be considered when children have digestive problems after experiencing grief or anxiety; typically, they have painless, urgent diarrhea. The child feels a lump or heaviness in the stomach. He may also have an empty feeling that is relieved by eating. Strangely enough, the nausea is sometimes ameliorated by eating. The child tends to have a peculiar appetite: averse to ordinary foods, warm food, and meat, but craving exotic foods, sour foods, and foods that are difficult to digest. The child sometimes craves bread, especially rye bread. He avoids fruits, sweets, and cold drinks, and sometimes sweats during eating. He feels relief from taking a deep breath, and so tends to sigh frequently, taking deep breaths each time. This remedy is commonly given to bulimic or anorexic adolescent girls.

IPECAC: When children have a persistent nausea that is not relieved by vomiting, this medicine should be considered. Another distinguishing symptom is that the child has a clean tongue, despite disordered digestion. She has little thirst and feels disgust for food. She feels nauseated after eating, especially veal, pork, indigestible foods, rich foods, pastry, ice cream, or sweets. She has a sensation as though her stomach was empty and flaccid (a sense as though it were hanging down). There is excessive salivation. The abdomen is bloated and tender to the touch. *Pulsatilla* is often preferred for nausea and vomiting when there is food in the stomach (if the child has other *Pulsatilla* symptoms), while *Ipecac* is more often indicated when the stomach is relatively empty.

Iris: A combination of headache with nausea, vomiting, and diarrhea (or constipation) typifies this medicine. The vomit is sour and acidic, commonly with a taste of vinegar. The child has a great deal of saliva and a burning of the whole digestive system (see Headaches).

Lycopodium: When children have gas and feel bloated after anything they eat they tend to need *Lycopodium*. They don't

INDIGESTION.

like belts or any type of tight pants due to the pressure exerted on their bloated abdomens. They typically experience the worst bloating between 4:00 P.M. and 8:00 P.M. Warm drinks provide some relief, and they are particularly aggravated by cold drinks, oysters, milk, peas, beans, cabbage, and pastry.

NUX VOMICA: This medicine should be considered when a child has a digestive upset after prolonged mental or emotional stress or after overindulging in food, alcohol, or drugs (either by the child or the breast-feeding mother). The child may want to vomit but has difficulty and instead retches frequently; if he is able to vomit, it provides relief. The child also suffers from distension of the abdomen, which is tender to the touch; he usually needs to loosen his pants. He is also very flatulent and feels better if he is able to pass gas. He tends to have heartburn, be bloated and gassy, and constipated with constant, futile attempts to pass a stool and a sense of never being finished. These children are irritable, and they often have headaches concurrent with their digestive problems.

PHOSPHORUS: Burning pains in the stomach that accompany nausea, vomiting, or diarrhea are characteristic of children who need this remedy. They feel worse after warm drinks or food and want cold drinks; however, these lead to nausea and vomiting once they warm in their stomachs. There is a sense of emptiness in the stomach, worse at night before bedtime when the child becomes very hungry. He is generally weak, anxious, and restless.

PULSATILLA: This medicine is invaluable for children who are *Pulsatilla* types (see "General Characteristics" in part 4) or for those who develop digestive problems after eating too much fruit, or greasy or rich foods. The child is also apt to develop digestive problems after ingesting cold or iced food or drinks, after exposure to cold, or after being emotionally upset. He develops his worst bloating and nausea at night, especially after dinner. The stools are changeable—sometimes watery,

INDIGESTION

sometimes formed, and sometimes formed in changing ways. Infants tend to have watery greenish diarrhea at night. The child feels chilly, though he is averse to warm or stuffy rooms and prefers cool and open air. The nausea is aggravated in a warm room. The child also benefits from walking slowly in the open air. He tends to be indecisive about what he wants to eat. He burps frequently.

Sepia: The child's nausea is usually worse in the morning and is accompanied by a sinking emptiness in the pit of the stomach. She is nauseated even by the smell of food. She wants sour things, such as pickles and vinegar, despite the nausea. She may also crave spicy things and sweets and will reject meat, fats, and milk. Fats, milk, and bread may aggravate the child's digestive problems.

INFLUENZA

Children with fevers higher than 103.5 degrees (taken orally) that do not respond to the above remedies or general home care within six hours should be given prompt medical care. Infants less than six months old should receive medical care for any fever higher than 100.5 degrees. Infants less than two months old should receive medical care for any fever. Also, when a child has any fever with extreme irritability, lethargy, and mental confusion along with stiffness of the neck, seizures, recurrent vomiting, or labored breathing, seek medical care immediately.

ACONITUM: This medicine should only be considered within twenty-four hours of the onset of symptoms. The child has a sudden onset of fever with chills. He is easily chilled when uncovered and gets the chills shortly after getting in bed. He has a rapid, hard pulse, and either a flushed face or one that alternates between being pale and being red.

ANAS BARBARIAE: Controlled scientific studies have proven this remedy effective in treating the flu. It is particularly effective if it is taken during the first forty-eight hours of the onset of the flu. Some homeopaths consider it a generic homeopathic remedy for the flu, while others find that it is primarily helpful when the flu has a rapid onset, causes a bursting headache, a painful cough, or when flu symptoms begin after the child has been exposed to a cold wind.

Arsenicum: A high fever comes on rapidly, along with a weak but restless feeling. The child is likely to have a concurrent headache, cold, sore throat, digestive disorder, or, most commonly, diarrhea. He is very thirsty but only for sips of water at a time. He is very chilly.

BELLADONNA: A distinguishing symptom of children who need this medicine is a flushed face and reddened mucous membranes, especially lips and gums. There is a sudden onset of high fever with a hot head and cold extremities. You can feel a radiating heat from the child's head. She feels dry and hot (without perspiration), has a strong and bounding pulse, and may hallucinate when her eyes are closed. She tosses and turns in her sleep and may have scary dreams.

BRYONIA: The fever has a slow onset and is typified by body aches which are worsened by motion. The child has a dry mouth and is thirsty for cold drinks. He is aggravated by warm rooms and warmth and prefers cool rooms and open air. He tends to have a headache in the front part of the head which is made worse by any motion. He is irritable and is averse to sympathy.

Eupatorium perfoliatum: A characteristic symptom of children who need this remedy is aching in the bones which is worse from motion. These children may experience chills at any time, but their chills tend to be worst in the morning between 7:00 A.M. and 9:00 A.M. and are preceded by thirst and great soreness, especially of their backs. Despite their chilliness, they crave cold drinks and even ice cream.

Ferrum phos: This medicine is primarily for the first stage of fever. The fever does not have the suddenness or intensity related to *Aconitum* or *Belladonna,* nor the degree of weariness associated with *Gelsemium* or the irritability characteristic of *Bryonia.*

GELSEMIUM: This is one of the most common medicines for influenza. The child suffers from great weakness and heaviness of the body; sometimes he is only able to open his eyes halfway because even his eyelids feel heavy. There is a general achiness and a headache in the back of the head. He avoids motion, not necessarily because it hurts to move but mostly because he feels so weak that motion exhausts him. He is also chilly and tries to stay warm. One of the unique symptoms is a sense of relief after urination. Another characteristic symptom is lack of thirst. This medicine is also commonly effective for children who have lingering symptoms, especially fatigue, after having the flu.

INFLUENZINUM: This remedy can be taken once a month (30x) during the flu season as a preventative. It is also helpful if a child has symptoms that linger after having the flu.

Rhus tox: These children experience achiness and stiffness that is aggravated by rest or by initial motion and relieved by continued motion. Because of this relief from continued motion, they seem restless and toss and turn. Their fever and aches become worse at night and in bed. In addition to stiffness in the back or neck, they may feel aching in the bones. The child may also have a dry cough or sneezing which is aggravated by cold or by being uncovered. Fever may alternate with chills. A rare but important keynote symptom is a tongue that is bright red at the tip.

INFLUENZA

INSECT BITES AND STINGS
See Bites and Stings.

INSOMNIA

Homeopathic medicines are often effective in treating the acute symptoms of insomnia, though professional constitutional care is usually necessary to achieve a deeper level of cure when this condition is chronic.

Aconitum: These children have difficulty falling and staying asleep due to fever and anxious dreaming. They are restless, and toss and turn in bed.

Argentum nit: The child is in a state of perpetual agitation, particularly just before bedtime. These children do things hurriedly, act impulsively, are restless, and seem to be driven. Sleep is disturbed by scary dreams, and they have great difficulty falling asleep if the room is too warm.

ARSENICUM: Various symptoms of the illness are aggravated at or after midnight. The child is both mentally and physically restless. She is anxious, fearful, and has scary dreams. The child tends to be very demanding of her parents, frequently yelling for their help. She is thirsty, but takes only sips of water at a time. She is chilly and does whatever she can to avoid being uncovered.

Chamomilla: The child has difficulty falling or staying asleep due to extreme irritability or due to the extreme pain he may be in. He demands things but refuses them once they are offered. He is sleepy but cannot sleep. He is temporarily relieved by being carried and rocked. He throws off the covers and may moan and twitch in his sleep.

COFFEA: This is one of the first remedies to consider for sleeplessness, expecially for children who are mentally hyperactive with a constant flow of ideas or plans for the next day. They are easily excitable. Sometimes the child's sleeplessness is the result of good news he recently received, and his excitable state makes it difficult for him to fall asleep. He also tends to be hypersensitive to sound. This is a good remedy for a breast-feeding infant whose mother drinks coffee.

IGNATIA: The most distinguishing symptom of children who need this medicine is frequent yawning. The cause of the insomnia is usually grief. The child sleeps very lightly and is distracted by the slightest noise. The extremities may jerk during sleep; there is a tendency to excessive dreaming.

KALI PHOSPHORICUM: When a child wakes with night terrors and then has difficulty falling asleep again, this remedy is indicated. Most typically, the child wakes screaming, is anxious, easily startled and restless, with particularly fidgety feet. He has constant thoughts and various anxieties, not only about nightmares but also about recent events in his life.

NUX VOMICA: Anxieties crowd these children's thoughts. They are worried and irritable. They tend to have dreams about school or quarrels. They are sensitive to any noise and are irritated by the slightest disturbance. They wake up at 3:00 A.M. or 4:00 A.M. and have difficulty falling back to sleep. They may have insomnia as a side effect of a medical drug.

Pulsatilla: The child resists going to sleep because she resists anything that separates her from her parents. She is impressionable and may have difficulty falling asleep if she is told a scary bedtime story or if anything else emotionally disturbing occurs shortly before bedtime. She tends to have repeated thoughts. She has a fear of being alone in the dark and will often get up and go to her parents' bed in the middle of the night. She may even have nightmares about her parents leaving her. She prefers and sometimes needs to have a light on in her room. The child likes to be rocked to sleep and tends to sleep with her hands above her head. Her insomnia is aggra-

INSOMNIA

vated by warm or stuffy rooms; she dislikes covers and usually kicks them off. She then tends to wake up because she is too cold.

RHUS TOX: The child's sleep is hindered by restlessness. Since her pain is lessened by continued motion, the child is aggravated by lying down and trying to sleep. She can't find a comfortable position, and she tosses and turns during sleep as well. She may get up in the middle of the night and feel stiff, will have pains upon first moving again, and less pain the more she moves.

STRAMONIUM: When a child wakes frequently in the middle of night full of terror, this medicine should be considered. He may also twitch and have convulsions during sleep, as well as hallucinations—such as seeing ghosts, animals, or even the Devil.

Staphysagria: This medicine should be considered when a child has difficulty falling asleep due to a highly emotional state in which she is brooding on past events—especially if her pride has been hurt or her emotions have been suppressed. It is a common medicine for abused children. These children are very sleepy in the afternoon with frequent yawning and stretching. They tend to have frightful dreams.

JET LAG

ARNICA: *Arnica* is the most commonly used homeopathic medicine for jet lag.

COCCULUS: Consider this remedy when a child feels slightly confused, spaced-out, or dizzy.

Gelsemium: When children are anxious, nervous, exhausted, or even tremble, this medicine should be given.

LARYNGITIS

Aconitum: This medicine is recommended for a child who develops laryngitis after exposure to cold. He may also have a dry cough.

Allium cepa: Hoarseness during a cold is an indication to use this medicine, especially if the nasal discharge is clear and watery.

Argenticum nit: This medicine is helpful for children who tend to be nervous, restless, and always on the move. They may get laryngitis from singing, talking, or yelling too much.

CAUSTICUM: A child who overuses her voice is most apt to benefit from this remedy. It is also the most common remedy to be given to children who are nervous prior to a performance or exam.

Hepar sulphur: Great hoarseness with a barking cough typifies children who need this medicine. They are apt to have gotten their hoarseness after being exposed to the cold or during heat. The symptoms are worse in the mornings. The child may also have a sore throat with pains extending to the ear when swallowing.

Kali bic: The distinguishing symptom is stringy, ropy yellow mucus that is coughed up. The child is prone to have a cold at the time and needs to hawk up mucus frequently. He has a sensation of a hair in the back of his throat. The hoarseness is worse after eating, drinking, being uncovered, or during cold weather, and is relieved by warmth and lying down in a warm bed.

PHOSPHORUS: The child has a dry cough and suffers from a scraping and burning pain in the throat, with a need to cough up mucus in the morning. Typically, a cold is concurrent with the hoarseness. The child craves and is relieved by ice drinks.

LARYNGITIS

MEASLES

Homeopathic medicines are often effective in treating measles, though medical attention should also be sought due to the possibility of complications from this disease.

ACONITUM: Useful at the beginning stages of measles. The child has a high fever, a dry barking cough, and reddened conjunctivas (pink eye). His skin burns and itches, and he feels restless, anxious, and frightened. He tosses and turns.

Apis: In these cases the rash begins but fails to develop fully, then soon disappears—though the child doesn't feel completely well. The itching is made worse by warmth, and the face and eyelids are puffy.

BELLADONNA: This remedy is often useful at the beginning stages of the measles when there is a sudden onset of high fever, a reddened face, and a throbbing headache. The child tends to be drowsy, a little delirious, and has some difficulty falling or staying asleep. Despite fever, she is not very thirsty.

Bryonia: In these cases the skin eruptions from the measles are delayed. The child has a hard, dry cough with no expectoration. Any motion causes pain. He may experience some mild delirium.

Euphrasia: The child has a fever and rash as well as acrid tears and a bland nasal discharge. He is sensitive to light. He has a cough, but only during the day.

Gelsemium: The onset of symptoms is slow. There is fever, great weakness, and a sense of heaviness, both of the whole body and specifically the eyelids. There is no thirst.

Kali bic: The child has a ropy, stringy discharge from the nose and burning, tearing eyes. Her salivary glands are noticeably swollen, and she may have stitching pains that go from the ear into the head and neck.

PULSATILLA: These children experience mild cases of the measles. Their fevers are not high, and their symptoms are not too painful. The child will, however, have profuse tearing from the eyes and considerable nasal discharge. He also has a dry cough at night which becomes loose in the daytime. He may have an ear inflammation. Although he has a dry mouth, he isn't thirsty.

Sulphur: The child has a purplish appearance. Her itching is aggravated by scratching. She has reddened mucous membranes and is very thirsty. Her cough and diarrhea are at their worst in the morning.

~

MOTION SICKNESS

Borax: The child has a fear of or gets sick from downward motion, such as during airplane landings or the pitching of a ship.

COCCULUS: This is one of the primary remedies for various types of travel sickness, whether it be from traveling in a car, boat, or airplane. The child feels dizzy and nauseous, and different from the child helped by *Tabacum,* he is worse in the fresh air. He is also worse after eating or drinking and may feel some relief when lying down. He may have a sense of emptiness or hollowness in his head or stomach. He may also tremble.

Petroleum: The child feels dizzy on rising, nauseous, and has a sinking feeling in the stomach. He may also get a headache in the back of the head. The symptoms tend to be worse in the fresh air.

Sepia: When children get motion sickness primarily from reading while traveling, consider this medicine.

MOTION SICKNESS

TABACUM: Along with dizziness and nausea, the child feels cold, faint, sweats, and has a sinking feeling in the stomach. She may experience some relief after vomiting. She may also be relieved by being in the open air; she feels worse in a stuffy room. A rare but helpful symptom to determine the appropriateness of giving *Tabacum* is if the child feels some relief from the nausea by baring her abdomen.

MUMPS

Homeopathic medicines are often effective in treating the average case of mumps and help reduce the chances of complications. However, any teenager who gets the mumps should receive medical attention, and so should any child who also has difficulty hearing or who has convulsions, neck stiffness, severe headache, or great weakness.

Aconitum: This is useful at the beginning stages of mumps. These children have a sudden onset of fever, and are restless, anxious, and very thirsty.

BELLADONNA: The child has a flushed face and a throbbing headache. He has swollen glands that are hot to touch. He is drowsy but has difficulty sleeping.

Mercurius: Right-sided swelling of throat glands typifies children who will benefit from this medicine. The child also has profuse and foul-smelling salivation and perspiration.

PHYTOLACCA: When a child with mumps has stony-hard throat glands, especially on the right side, this medicine should be considered. The throat pains may extend to the ear, and the child may have an irresistible desire to clamp his teeth together. One of the characteristic symptoms is pain from sticking out the tongue. The child tends to be worse in cold or wet weather.

MUMPS

PILOCARPINUM: Some homeopaths assert that this medicine is the best remedy for the mumps, although there are few known distinguishing symptoms that indicate it, except excessive salivation and perspiration. This is also a good remedy for the complications that some children get from the mumps.

Pulsatilla: This medicine is helpful for a child approaching puberty who gets the mumps and has swollen breasts or testicles. The child has no thirst, despite the fever, and is sensitive to warm rooms.

Rhus tox: These children have swollen glands which are worse on the left side. Their symptoms are aggravated by cold, and they may have cold sores on their lips.

MUSCLE INJURIES

ARNICA: This medicine—taken internally as well as applied externally—is effective in treating muscle pain from injury or overexertion. It is also good for old injuries that are still bothersome.

Bellis perennis: When there are bumps or lumps remaining after an injury, this medicine should be given.

NAUSEA AND VOMITING
See Food Poisoning or Indigestion.

NERVE INJURIES
See also Smashed Fingers or Toes.

Nerve injuries can be serious. Seek medical attention if there is numbness or loss of sensation.

NERVE INJURIES

HYPERICUM: This is the primary medicine for injuries to nerves or to parts of the body rich with nerves: crushed fingers or toes, falls injuring the spine, blows to the head, or injury to the front teeth or tongue. If a child experiences convulsions after a head injury, this is the first medicine to consider on the way to seeking professional medical care. It is also helpful for phantom limb pains, twitching, or any neurological complaint after an injury.

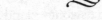

NERVOUS RESTLESSNESS

Homeopathic medicine is often effective in treating the acute symptoms of nervous restlessness, though professional constitutional care is usually necessary to cure a chronic hyperactive state.

ARGENTUM NIT: These children are in a state of perpetual agitation. They do things hurriedly, act impulsively, are restless, and driven; they generate an atmosphere of turbulence. They are anxious about their health and about upcoming engagements. They have a strong craving for sweets, yet they tend to be worse from them. The child's body is warm and is aggravated by heat.

ARSENICUM: The child is very restless, high-strung and nervous, and easily prone to fright. He tends to be anxious all the time, whether it is about something specific or just a generalized anxious feeling. He feels compelled to move from bed to chair, chair to bed, and room to room. Mentally, he is afraid of increased troubles. He thinks that his problem is much more serious than it actually is. He may repeatedly ask his parents what is wrong with him. He is fastidious, and this anxious and fussy meticulousness will compel him to clean his room, even when he feels quite ill. He is easily frightened and is particularly scared of being alone and being in the dark. His vivid imagination conjures up creative fears and his restlessness takes him out of his own bed and into his parents'.

CHAMOMILLA: Particularly common for restless infants, this medicine is helpful when the infant also throws temper tantrums. She asks for things but then refuses them once they are offered. Nothing satisfies her, though carrying and rocking provide short-term relief.

Coffea: This remedy is good for breast-feeding infants whose mothers drink coffee, or for children who are hurried in their motions, their eating and drinking, their speech, and their play. These children are physically and mentally restless.

NUX VOMICA: Used for children who are hyperactive and overexcitable. They tend to throw tantrums at home or in public, and then wildly fend off anyone who tries to stop them. They thrive on rebellion. The child's revved-up nervous system makes him oversensitive to touch, pain, noise, odors, music, food, and drugs. He is a light sleeper, easily woken, and gets angry at whoever woke him up.

Rhus tox: The child is physically and psychologically restless. She is always on the move and feels uneasy staying in one position. She is particularly restless at night and will toss and turn in bed. She becomes confused and tends to forget where or why she is going somewhere.

NOSEBLEEDS
See Bleeding.

~

POISON IVY OR OAK

ANACARDIUM: This remedy is given to children with poison ivy or poison oak when they feel excessive itching and burning, which increases after scratching. The child becomes irritable. He uses violent language, even if he usually doesn't when he's healthy. He becomes absent-minded. The eruptions tend to occur on the face (though this medicine may still provide relief even if this is not the case). Rubbing and eating may provide temporary relief. The child may get some relief from applications of hot water but a hot bath makes him feel worse. There may be redness around the pustules.

Croton tig: Intense itching leads the child to hard scratching which causes increased burning, while light scratching or gentle rubbing provide some relief. The skin feels tight and hidebound—a feeling temporarily relieved after sleep. The medicine is particularly helpful for rashes on the face and genitals, though it is not limited to these areas. Typically the skin is very red, sometimes scarlet. The eruptions will have small blisters which ooze and dry into yellow scabs.

Graphites: The distinguishing symptom of children who need this remedy is skin eruptions that exude a thick, glutinous, sticky, honey-colored fluid. The skin areas around a joint and parts usually covered by clothing are the most frequently affected. The itching can be severe, accompanied by burning and stinging, usually worse at night, from heat, and after exposure to water.

LEDUM: A skin rash that itches and is relieved by cold water or cold applications is an indication to use this medicine. It can also be used shortly after exposure to poison oak or ivy as a way to prevent a rash from developing.

RHUS TOX: Consider this remedy when the child has skin eruptions that itch and burn and when scratching does not provide relief but actually increases the irritation. The rash stings and burns and is aggravated at night and by warmth of bed. Bathing tends to worsen the condition, though hot water, especially scalding water, as well as warm applications are soothing. The skin eruptions may have pus in them and sometimes erupt in a line of a previous scratch. Some homeopaths

POISON IVY OR OAK

suggest that the 3x or 6x are the most effective potencies for treating this condition.

Sepia: These children do not get relief from scratching. Their overall skin coloring tends to be of a sallow, yellowish tinge.

SULPHUR: The child's rash burns and itches and is worsened by warm bathing. Warmth, especially the warmth of bed, aggravates the condition. Scratching feels good but usually causes increased burning. The child may be so driven to scratch the eruptions that he scratches them until they bleed.

PUNCTURE WOUNDS

Any wound that is deep or dirty (such as stepping on a rusty nail) requires medical attention.

LEDUM: This is the primary remedy for puncture wounds. The wound is worse by warmth, especially the warmth of bed, and is relieved by applications of cold or ice. The wound is very sensitive to touch.

STAPHYSAGRIA: This medicine is more often given for deeper puncture wounds or stabs, especially those affecting organs.

SCARS

Homeopathic medicines can sometimes reduce the degree of scarring that children experience.

CALENDULA: The tincture (undiluted), gel, spray, or oil should be directly applied to the scar and surrounding tissue.

GRAPHITES: This is the primary remedy for injury-induced keloids (a fibrous tumor that forms a hard, irregularly shaped eruption on the skin). *Graphites* is taken internally.

SCARS

~

SHOCK FROM INJURY

Shock can be treated homeopathically, but children suffering from severe shock should also receive medical attention. If a child has a rapid heart rate, shallow, irregular breathing, and is confused or unconscious, medical care is essential.

<u>ACONITUM</u>: If a child is very restless, anxious, and fearful, give this medicine.

<u>ARNICA</u>: *Arnica* is the primary remedy to consider for shock from injury. *Arnica* is more useful when the child is traumatized by the pain or confused as to the extent of the injury, while *Aconitum* is more useful when the child is primarily suffering emotional shock along with the physical pain.

~

SINUSITIS

Homeopathic medicines are often effective in treating the acute symptoms of sinusitis, although professional constitutional care is usually necessary to cure chronic sinusitis.

Arsenicum: The child feels throbbing and burning pains in the sinuses which are aggravated by light, noise, movement, after midnight, and may be triggered by anxiety, exertion, and excitement. The child may feel relief by lying quietly in a dark room with the head raised on pillows and exposed to cool air. The teeth may feel long and painful. There may be nausea and vomiting concurrent with the sinusitis.

<u>BELLADONNA</u>: There are throbbing pains in the front part of the head that come on suddenly and tend to leave suddenly only to return (see Headaches).

<u>HEPAR SULPHUR</u>: This is rarely used at the beginning of a sinusitis condition. The child begins sneezing and then develops

sinusitis from the least exposure to cold air. The nasal discharge is thick and yellow. The nostrils become very sore from the acrid discharge, and the nasal passages become sensitive to cold air. The child may also have a headache with a sense of a nail or a plug that is thrust into the head—a boring or bursting pain. The headache above the nose is worse from shaking the head, motion, riding in a car, stooping, moving the eyes, or simply from the weight of a hat, but is relieved by the firm pressure of a tight bandage. The scalp is so sensitive that even combing the child's hair may be painful.

KALI BIC: The distinguishing feature of children with sinusitis who need this medicine is that they have a thick, stringy nasal discharge. There is extreme pain at the root of the nose that is better when pressure is applied there. The bones and scalp feel sore. Dizziness and nausea when rising from sitting and severe pain may lead to dimmed vision. The pains are made worse by cold, light, noise, walking, stooping, and are bad in the morning (especially on waking or at 9 A.M.) or at night. The child prefers to lie down in a darkened room and feels better when warm, when given warm drinks, or when he overeats.

Mercurius: The child feels as though her head was in a vise. The pains are worse in open air, from sleeping, and after eating and drinking. The pains are also aggravated by extremes of hot and cold. The scalp and the nose become very sensitive to touch. The teeth feel long and painful, and the child may salivate excessively. The nasal discharge is usually green and too thick to run. It is offensive-smelling and acrid.

PULSATILLA: The head pain is worse when the child lies down and is in a warm room; it is better in cool air. The sinusitis may begin after the child is overheated. Stooping, sitting, rising from lying down, and eating can aggravate the head pain, which is often in the front part of the head and accompanied by digestive problems. The child feels relief walking slowly in

SINUSITIS

the open air or by having her head wrapped tightly in a bandage. This condition is commonly experienced when the child is in school. The nasal discharge is often thick and yellow or green.

<u>Silicea:</u> The child usually has a chronically stuffed nose. He feels as if his head will burst. The head pain tends to be worse in one eye, usually the right. It is aggravated by mental exertion (students tend to get sinusitis while studying for an exam). Cold air, moving the head, light, or noise can also aggravate the head pain. It is relieved by wrapping the head warmly and tightly or by applying heat.

<u>Spigella:</u> Children who develop sinusitis with a sharp pain that is worse on the left side may need this medicine. They tend to get sinusitis after exposure to cold or wet weather. They feel pain from warmth or when they stoop or bend the head forward, and they feel some relief by cold applications or from washing with cold water.

∼

SMASHED FINGERS OR TOES

<u>Arnica:</u> Use this remedy for the initial shock of injury and to help the body reabsorb the blood that has pooled under the skin. (Use *Hypericum* as well, which helps speed the process of healing.)

<u>HYPERICUM:</u> This medicine helps to reduce the sharp or shooting pains from injuries and to begin the healing of any damaged nerves.

∼

SORE THROAT

Homeopathic medicines are often effective in treating the acute symptoms of a sore throat, though professional constitutional care is usually necessary to cure chronically recurring sore throats. A child with much pain from a sore throat or one who has difficulty opening his mouth or swallowing should have a culture taken to determine if he has strep.

ACONITUM: Consider this medicine during the onset of the sore throat. The symptoms come on suddenly, often after exposure to cold air. There may be some burning in the throat and a red, dry, swollen throat.

APIS: The child has a red, inflamed throat with swollen tonsils, which is aggravated by warm drinks or food and relieved by cold drinks and sucking on an ice cube. This remedy should be considered when the throat hurts even when the child isn't swallowing. The throat not only looks red, it looks shiny. There is dryness in the throat with a burning, stinging pain. The child has a constrictive feeling in the throat. The inner and outer throat is swollen, and the uvula which hangs from the upper throat is also swollen. The child may have a sensation of a fishbone caught in the throat and may have difficulty swallowing. He may be hoarse in the mornings and cannot stand to have anything around his neck.

Arsenicum: Consider this medicine when the child has a burning pain in the throat that is relieved by warm food or drinks and aggravated by cold food or drinks. The condition may begin with a nasal discharge and then go into the throat. The pains are usually worse on the right side. The mouth may also be dry, and there is great thirst for frequent sips of water.

BELLADONNA: This medicine is the most common remedy for acute tonsillitis. It is also commonly given at the early stages of other types of sore throat. The tonsils are noticeably red, usually scarlet red. There are burning pains and a constant desire to swallow, despite the fact that it hurts to do so. There is a constricted feeling in the throat, which causes difficulty swallowing—even swallowing water. The child wants lemons or lemonade. There is a tickling in the larnyx. If the

SORE THROAT

child has a fever, it will usually be a high one. Characteristically, the head is hot, though the extremities are cold.

Ferrum phos: This remedy is common for acute, nonviolent tonsillitis. The inflammation does not begin suddenly, and the pain is not severe. The throat is red and swollen, especially on waking. It is painful to swallow, usually a burning pain, which feels better when cold is applied. The child may also be hoarse. This remedy is helpful for the child who sings a lot, and seems to get a sore throat because of it.

Hepar sulphur: When a child has a sensation as though there was a stick in his throat, or when a sore throat starts after the child is exposed to cold, this medicine should be considered. The tonsils are enlarged, and they throb painfully. Swallowing creates a pain that radiates to the ears. Hot drinks provide some relief. These children are hypersensitive to touch and cold and are highly irritable.

Ignatia: The distinguishing symptom is sore throat pain that is relieved by swallowing foods and is aggravated by empty swallowing. (*Lachesis* also addresses this symptom.) The child may have throat pain even when she doesn't swallow. She tends to have a lump in her throat, sometimes related to the suppression of some strong emotion. Sometimes she is hoarse or loses her voice completely. She is highly emotional—evidenced by her tendency to take deep breaths or to sigh frequently.

LACHESIS: When children have a sore throat that is worse on the left side, this medicine is often indicated. The left gland in the throat is more swollen, and inside the throat the left side is more red, sometimes purplish. There is a feeling of a constant tickle or of a fishbone caught in the throat. The pains are worsened by empty swallowing (just swallowing saliva) or drinking warm or hot liquids; the pains are eased by swallowing foods. The throat particularly hurts when the child tries to cough up mucus. The throat is hypersensitive to touch, which

SORE THROAT

explains why the child does not like wearing clothes with tight collars.

Lycopodium: This medicine should be considered when the child has a sore throat that is worse on the right side or that starts on the right and moves to the left. Although the child may not notice the difference, if you look in the throat you will be able to see more inflammation on one side or the other. The pain is aggravated by swallowing cold liquids and relieved by warm ones. The child may feel a choking sensation, as though a ball was stuck in her throat.

MERCURIUS: This child has a cold that settles in his throat. He wants to swallow constantly and feels a lot of pain every time he does. In extreme cases, he has a choking sensation on swallowing. There is much redness and swelling in the throat along with a raw, burning pain. The throat is dry despite a great deal of saliva in the mouth. There may be so much salivation that the child needs to swallow frequently, and he may wet his pillow with it. He has swollen tonsils and lymph glands, and his throat pain extends to his ear. The throat may be ulcerated and tends to be worse on the right side. Another characteristic symptom is noticeably bad breath. When a child has these symptoms along with a left-sided sore throat, give *Mercurius iodatus ruber;* when a child has a right-sided sore throat, give *Mercurius iodatus flavus.*

Phytolacca: There are two types of pain that are experienced when swallowing which are characteristic of the need for this medicine: shooting pain from the throat into the ears, and pain at the root of the tongue that causes pain when the child sticks out her tongue. She has a feeling of rawness and roughness in the throat, which is usually worse on the right side and while drinking hot fluids. The child feels a swollen, constricted feeling in the throat. The tonsils tend to be swollen and may have been swollen for a long time. The glands in the neck are also swollen.

SORE THROAT

RHUS TOX: These children have throat pain on initial swallowing but experience relief the more often they swallow.

Sulphur: This medicine is helpful for children who have burning pains in their throats that are aggravated by warm food or drinks and relieved by cold drinks. They have swollen tonsils and offensive breath.

Wyethia: When a child has a tickling sensation on the roof of his mouth or in the throat that stimulates coughing, this medicine should be considered. Another important indication for this medicine is a sore throat caused by an allergy. It is also effective in treating sore throats in the child who sings a lot or who irritates his throat from overuse. He usually has a dry, hot, and swollen throat with a constant desire to swallow saliva, despite having difficulty swallowing.

SPLINTERS

Homeopathic medicines can help remove splinters which have become deeply imbedded into the skin. The correct remedy seems to strengthen the body's efforts to push out the foreign substance.

HEPAR SULPHUR: If *Silicea* does not work, consider giving this medicine for imbedded splinters that cannot be easily removed with tweezers.

SILICEA: *Silicea* is the primary remedy for helping the body expel splinters or any foreign object trapped under the skin.

SPRAINS AND STRAINS

ARNICA: This is the first remedy to give for sprains and strains from injury or overexertion. Other remedies should be given after *Arnica*.

SPRAINS AND STRAINS

Bellis perennis: When children have severe sprains, consider giving this medicine.

Bryonia: When *Arnica* or *Rhus tox* are not working well enough to heal a sprain, give this medicine. It is also effective in treating the pain of this kind of injury (which is worse with any motion).

Ledum: Children who easily sprain their ankles can benefit from taking this medicine.

RHUS TOX: This is the primary medicine for sprains. While *Arnica* is helpful at first to keep the swelling down, *Rhus tox* helps heal the sprain itself. The injury typically feels stiff and painful; it is worse on initial motion and loosens up from continued motion. It is also good for sprains or strains from overexertion, especially of muscles that are not frequently used.

RUTA: Severe strains in which a child wrenches or tears a tendon may be helped by this medicine. The injured part will feel hot to the touch. The British often alternate between *Arnica* and *Ruta.*

STOMACH CRAMPS. See Colic.

STYES

Apis: This medicine is effective when tears burn and there is puffiness of the eyelid that is worse by heat and better by cold applications.

BELLADONNA: The stye comes on very quickly. The eye is red and dry. The child tends to be sensitive to light and have dilated pupils.

PULSATILLA: The styes are recurrent and are aggravated by warm applications and relieved by cold applications. The

STYES

child tends to get styes on the upper lid, and sometimes there is a yellowish or green-yellowish discharge.

Staphysagria: Like children who need *Pulsatilla,* these children get recurrent styes, though they tend to have more itching at the edges of their eyelids.

Sulphur: There are hot, burning pains aggravated by heat and bathing. Any discharge from the eye tends to burn the surrounding skin.

SUNBURN. See Burns.

SURGERY

These medicines are valuable in helping the child's body adapt to the shock caused by surgery and in helping to speed the healing process. Some of the medicines are useful in reducing the potential problems from radiation used as a diagnostic aid through X-rays or as a treatment of certain cancers. Professional homeopathic care will inevitably be a useful adjunct to treat the condition for which the child is having surgery.

Aconitum: When the child is fearful, anxious, and restless prior to or after surgery, this medicine should be considered.

ARNICA: This is the best medicine for physiological shock or trauma from surgery.

Bellis perennis: This medicine is helpful before or after abdominal surgery.

Ginseng: Ginseng has been shown to reduce some of the side effects of radiation. Give three doses of either the 6th or 30th potency every four hours prior to radiation and every three hours for the subsequent two days.

SURGERY

HYPERICUM: This medicine is primarily helpful both before and after surgeries involving nerve tissue, such as surgery on the feet, hands, spine, eye, head, and any surgery that causes sharp or shooting pains. It is also invaluable for dental surgery when there are sharp or shooting pains.

RUTA: When children have surgery on bones or teeth, this medicine should be considered. It has also been shown to reduce some of the side effects of radiation. It is the remedy of choice before and after dental X-rays. Give three doses of the 30th potency every four hours prior to radiation and every three hours for the subsequent two days.

Staphysagria: This is the best medicine to give before and after abdominal surgery.

TEETHING

BELLADONNA: These babies experience great pain that makes them restless and may lead them to kick, scream, or bite. They have very red gums and lips, and they may twitch.

CALCAREA CARB: The infant begins teething late (after twelve months). The head perspires during teething, and the child tends to grind his teeth at night. He usually puts his fingers in his mouth to try to relieve the pain. His sweat, stools, and vomit will all have a sour smell.

Calcarea phos: This medicine is for thin, even emaciated, infants who are slow in learning to walk, delayed in teething (after twelve months), and in general are slow starters. They are prone to diarrhea with much flatulence during teething.

CHAMOMILLA: This is the first medicine to consider, unless some other remedy is obviously indicated. The baby is extremely irritable and impatient. She demands something and then refuses it when it is offered. She seems to be in great pain. She is aggravated by being touched, and nothing seems to give her relief, though rocking and being carried temporarily quiets her. She puts her fingers in her mouth to relieve the pain. One cheek is often hot and red (the side of the inflamed gum), while the other cheek is cold and pale. She is relieved slightly by cold applications (ice). She has difficulty sleeping and will usually keep you up too. She may have green stools that smell like rotten eggs. Her arms or legs may jerk or convulse. If *Chamomilla* fails, it is usually best to try *Belladonna*.

Coffea: When teething infants are physically or mentally hyperactive and do not sleep much, consider this medicine.

Magnesia phos: These infants experience spasms during teething, which are relieved by warm or hot drinks.

Plantago: When an infant has ear pain concurrent with teething, take the tincture of this remedy and rub it directly on the gum, as well as placing a couple of slightly diluted drops into the ear.

THRUSH

Borax: The child has canker sores, white spots, and patches in his mouth. His mouth feels hot to the mother's nipple. The infant may experience so much pain from nursing that he refuses to nurse.

Hydrastis: When a child has thrush with a yellow-streaked tongue and expectoration of yellow mucus, consider this medicine.

Mercurius: When children have much salivation with their canker sores, this remedy should be considered. The canker sores may be in the mouth or on the tongue. The tongue is often noticeably moist and coated.

TOOTHACHE

Severe tooth pain should receive care from a dentist.

<u>Aconitum</u>: When children experience excruciating dental pain that makes them frantic, this medicine should be considered. The pains are usually worse at night and in cold temperatures, causing great restlessness and anxiety.

<u>ARNICA</u>: This medicine is good both before and after tooth extraction or any other dental surgery.

<u>BELLADONNA</u>: When there is rapid onset of throbbing pain that is better with warmth, this medicine is valuable. The gums are red and swollen; the child's face is flushed and the skin is hot. The child moans, especially when exposed to the air. He tends to have dilated pupils.

<u>Chamomilla</u>: The child is in extreme pain that is worse at night and made worse by warm applications or warm drinks and made better by cold things (she prefers to suck on an ice cube). She is extremely irritable. She cries loudly and persistently. Rocking and carrying her provides relief, but only temporarily.

<u>COFFEA</u>: The toothache makes the child extremely restless and sleepless. He feels some relief from cold water, while the pain is aggravated by warm drinks or food.

<u>HEPAR SULPHUR</u>: There is tooth pain from the slightest touch and from exposure to cold water, food, or air. These children are hyperirritable.

<u>HYPERICUM</u>: When children have shooting pains from injury or infection, this medicine should be considered. It is also good for injuries to the front teeth.

<u>Mercurius</u>: The child salivates profusely during a toothache.

The pains are aggravated by biting, cold air, and at night. They may extend to the ears.

Nux moschata: The child has severe throbbing pain that extends to neighboring teeth or to the ear. Usually the pains are aggravated by cold and relieved by warmth.

Plantago: Like children who need *Mercurius,* these children salivate a great deal with their toothaches. Their teeth are sensitive to touch and to extremes of temperature. They may experience some pain or twitching of their eyelids along with their toothaches.

RUTA: This medicine is beneficial before and after a tooth extraction.

Staphysagria: The tooth pain is so sensitive that the child cannot stand the slightest touch. The pains are worse from cold drinks or cold air.

X-RAY EXPOSURE

Ginseng: This medicine reduces some of the side effects of radiation. Give three doses of either the 6th or 30th potency every four hours prior to radiation and every three hours for the subsequent two days.

RUTA: This medicine has beneficial effects on bones and connective tissue, and also reduces some of the side effects of radiation. It is the remedy of choice before and after dental X-rays. Give three doses of the 30th potency every four hours prior to radiation and every three hours for the subsequent two days.

PART 4

Essential Homeopathic Medicines

This section of the book contains vital information about the most commonly given homeopathic medicines for children (the ones that were underlined in part 3). It not only provides more detailed information about these common remedies, it gives you a more detailed picture of the physical and psychological ailments that each medicine can successfully treat.

For instance, if your child has a sore throat, and you have read about the recommended medicines for this condition in part 3, you may have determined that *Aconitum* is the remedy that most closely fits your child's symptoms. However, after reading more in-depth information about *Aconitum* in part 4 and then reading more about another sore throat remedy, *Arsenicum*, you may realize that *Arsenicum* is the more accurately indicated remedy for your child.

The information in this section gives you a broader "portrait" of the various physical complaints and psychological characteristics that each remedy is known to treat. Reading part 4 not only increases your chances of finding the most effective medicine but also gives you valuable general information about specific medicines which may be useful in treating other health conditions your child may experience.

You will need to flip back and forth from part 3 to part 4 in order to get an overall sense of both the local symptoms and the general characteristics of the medicines. This extra effort will be rewarded by finding a more effective remedy and having a healthier child.

Do not expect a child to have all the symptoms listed under a medicine. Simply look for the medicine that most closely matches the *key* symptoms that the child is experiencing (you may want to reread part 2, which describes which symptoms are most important in choosing a medicine). Place more emphasis on the most intense symptoms. Also, place more emphasis on the symptoms that the child has at the moment. For instance, if your child normally likes drinks with ice in them but during this particular illness she craves warm drinks, then look for a medicine that describes a craving for warm drinks.

The description of the general characteristics of each medicine in this section includes the child's acute psychological symptoms and the constitutional characteristics (aspects of the child's personality) as well as the general physical symptoms (described in part 2 as those symptoms that affect the entire body rather than just parts of it). The correct remedy is sometimes based more on the general characteristics than the local symptoms about which the child is complaining. Making the decision on whether to place more emphasis on the general characteristics or the local symptoms may sometimes be difficult; however, priority is definitely given to the remedy that matches the child's general characteristics when at least one key physical symptom fits the child's condition.

Homeopaths will often place greater emphasis on the psychological symptoms than the physical symptoms for treating *chronic* illnesses, while such emphasis is sometimes but not always given priority in treating *acute* ailments. Psychological symptoms in acute ailments are primarily important when they are intense or obviously different than during the child's normal state.

Certain medicines are more often prescribed based upon their general characteristics than their local symptoms, notably *Calcarea carb, Chamomilla, Ignatia, Pulsatilla,* and *Sulphur.* If the general characteristics of a medicine fit your child, this medicine is often helpful in relieving a variety of acute and chronic health problems.

The medicines listed in part 4 are the most commonly used remedies in treating the health conditions of infants and children. Because of this, they should be an integral part of your home medicine kit. You should also add any medicines listed in part 3 which you think may be useful to you and your family.

Since homeopathic medicines are not often available in neighborhood pharmacies, it is worth purchasing a selection of at least thirty-five homeopathic medicines. Such advance preparation is invaluable; the medicines are already on hand and you are quickly able to help your children heal from the inevitable ailments and injuries to which they are prone. Most homeopathic companies sell medicine kits containing from twenty-eight to fifty ingredients. Homeopathic medicine kits are generally developed for health conditions of both children and adults, though some small medicine kits, consisting of six or so medicines, have been specifically developed for common childhood ailments.

Some medicine kits consist of remedies in the 6th potency, others in the 30th potency, and others in varying potencies. Those who want to be especially well-prepared have remedies in both the 6th and the 30th potency. It is generally recommended to use the higher potency (the 30th) when you are more certain about the accuracy of the remedy and to use the lower potency (the 6th) when you are not as confident. (See "Choosing the Correct Potency and Dose" in part 2 for further guidelines.)

Homeopathic manufacturers sell the medicine kits at special discount prices. Typically, over $100 worth of homeopathic medicines are available in a kit at less than half the cost of buying the medicines individually. Ideally, it is recommended to have a homeopathic medicine kit both at home, and (if you drive one) in the family car.

Various characteristics of each medicine are discussed in this chapter.

1. *Its Latin name and common names:* Because homeopathy is practiced throughout the world, its medicines must be known by the precise species of plant or animal used to create them. Hence, the formal Latin name for each medicine is given. An additional name is sometimes given after the formal Latin name; this is the abbreviated Latin name by which the medicine is usually referred to. One or more common names of the substance are also provided here; these are the names with which you will probably be more familiar.

2. *Overview:* General information about the specific plant, mineral, or animal is given; for example, what it looks and acts like in nature , or if it is used medicinally by physicians or healers other than homeopaths.

3. *General characteristics:* The general symptoms are described; that is, those physical and psychological symptoms that affect the whole child rather than local parts of his body (as discussed in part 2). These general symptoms help to characterize the type of child who would most benefit from this medicine. The general characteristics of a remedy are vital information and are the most important parts of this section.

4. *Keynote symptoms:* Keynote symptoms are those symptoms which are characteristic of children who would benefit from the medicine. Keynote symptoms can be either physical or psychological symptoms, local or general symptoms, or they could be modalities.

5. *Modalities:* Modalities are factors that aggravate or alleviate a child's overall health or specific pains.

6. *Primary indicated conditions:* Primary indicated conditions are those ailments which the medicine is known to treat. You will find the specific symptoms that this medicine treats listed under each of these conditions in part 3.

Armed with this information, you will be able to use homeopathic medicines more effectively. Not only will you feel better with this information, but so will your child.

~

ACONITUM/Aconite
(Common names: Aconite, Monkshood, Wolfsbane)

Overview

The herb aconite derives its name from the Greek work *akontion,* meaning "dart," because sharpened objects were dipped in its poisonous juices and then used to kill wolves or other animals that threatened people. Its juice is so poisonous that if it was applied to a wounded finger, the whole body would be affected, initially causing pains in the limbs, a sense of suffocation, and then fainting.

Aconite has been used in the East and the West for several centuries. Sidney Ringer (1835–1910), the famed British physician after whom the intravenous fluid *Ringer's Solution* is named, stated that "perhaps no drug is more valuable than aconite." However, because it contains a highly toxic alkaloid called *Aconitine,* which is a deadly poison, only small or specially prepared doses of this herb are used medicinally. Due to its ability to control inflammation and subdue accompanying fever, aconite became a very popular medicine used by American and European conventional physicians in the nineteenth century. However, it fell into disfavor among them because

ACONITUM/Aconite

they found that it was not consistently effective in treating fevers.

Homeopaths, on the other hand, used *Aconitum* much more successfully because they understood that this medicine, like all medicines, needed to be individually prescribed. Homeopaths found that *Aconitum* was a highly effective medicine when used to treat the unique pattern of symptoms that the herb aconite caused in healthy people.

Aconitum, in fact, is considered the vitamin C of homeopathy. It is primarily indicated at the initial stages of a high fever, acute inflammation (ear infection, respiratory infection, or sore throat) and shock from injury. It is rarely given to people for chronic or recurring symptoms.

General Characteristics

Aconitum is much more commonly used by laypeople than by medical professionals, primarily because the condition has usually progressed beyond the *Aconitum* stage by the time the sick person gets professional care.

A child who needs *Aconitum* typically has a sudden, sometimes intense onset of symptoms, usually coming shortly after exposure to cold, dry weather, especially if the child is perspiring at the time. Considering how often children develop colds, coughs, sore throats, or other common ailments after being exposed to cold, dry weather, *Aconitum* is an often-used remedy, though it is most effective if it is given within twenty-four hours of the onset of symptoms.

Parents who live in cold climates should expect to use *Aconitum* often. A sudden onset of symptoms may also follow exposure to extremely hot weather. This is why parents do their best to insist that their children be properly dressed. It's not that cold or heat actually causes illness; the extremes of weather stress the child's body enough so that his resistance is lowered, increasing the chances of getting ill if he is exposed to a virus or bacteria.

ACONITUM/Aconite

Varying degrees of restlessness, anxiety, and fear are shown by a child who needs *Aconitum,* depending upon the severity of the illness. Tossing and turning in bed is very common. He is irritated by noise or even music. He may also have foreboding feelings that his condition may worsen, and he may have a sense of urgency that something should be done to help him. In extreme cases, he may think that he is dying.

The child may feel a great deal of pain, which he describes as unbearable. The pain is aggravated by touch or when the child is uncovered.

The child's skin is hot and dry. The face will usually redden, though this flushing may alternate with pallor. The pulse is rapid and hard.

Aconitum is indicated at the initial stages of various inflammatory conditions and is usually not effective once pus or significant amounts of mucus are present.

Typically, the child who needs *Aconitum* has an intense thirst, usually for cold fluids. In some cases, he may have an unquenchable thirst.

A child who needs *Aconitum* may have difficulty falling asleep because his symptoms are most intense late at night. Hyperacute senses will also disturb his ability to fall asleep. His restlessness and pain prevent sound sleep.

The body experiences varying degrees of shock while undergoing surgery. *Aconitum* is often effective in reducing the fear and anxiety commonly experienced prior to and after surgery.

Keynote Symptoms

- The first stage of many infectious diseases

- Sudden onset of symptoms, especially after exposure to cold, dry wind

- Restlessness, anxiety, fear, feeling of foreboding

ACONITUM/Aconite

Modalities

Worse: dry, cold wind; warm rooms; evening and night; lying on the affected side; music.

Better: open air, after perspiring; when sitting still.

Primary Indicated Conditions

anxiety
asthma
black eye
bladder infection
bleeding
chickenpox
common cold
cough
croup
earache
eye injury
fever

German measles
hepatitis
indigestion
insomnia
influenza
laryngitis
measles
mumps
shock from injury
sore throat
surgery
toothache

ALLIUM CEPA
(Common name: Red onion)

Overview

When you cut an onion and get sprayed by its juices, you suddenly display the classic symptoms of the common cold: watery nasal discharge, watery eyes, and sneezing. These discharges, in the case of the cold, are the body's efforts to rid itself of the viruses which were killed by the white blood cells, many of which were killed themselves fighting the viral infection and which are also in the discharge. It is thus perfectly logical to use a medicine that stimulates mucus production to treat a person with a cold since this medicine will help the body flush out the dead virus and dead white blood cells.

ALLIUM CEPA

The ability of onions to dissolve mucus enables them to be an effective expectorant, helping the body clear the throat and chest of mucus. Onions are known to have natural antibiotic properties. Even scientist Louis Pasteur tested onions and observed their antibacterial activity. Present-day pulmonary specialist Dr. Irwin Ziment notes that eating raw onions can be helpful for throat and respiratory infections because onions release a "flood of tears" which helps to break up mucus congestion.

Dr. Victor Gurewich, a professor of medicine at Tufts University, has found that onions also stimulate the body's clot-dissolving abilities, thus improving cardiovascular health and helping blood circulation.

General Characteristics

Typically, exposure to the juice of an onion causes a profuse, watery nasal discharge and streaming watery eyes. More specifically, onions cause a burning nasal discharge that tends to irritate the nostrils and the upper lip. Children with colds who will benefit from *Allium cepa* are those who tend to complain that the tissue paper they use to blow their nose is too rough (despite it being as soft as it always is).

A child who needs *Allium cepa* will have reddened nostrils and upper lip and watery eyes. Sometimes you can simply look at a child with a cold and know that *Allium cepa* would be an effective medicine for them.

The child's eyes burn and may be tearing as much as her nose is dripping, but her tears will not be similarly acrid; thus her cheeks will not be irritated or reddened from the tears. Another homeopathic medicine, *Euphrasia* (eye-bright), is indicated when the child has the reverse symptoms of *Allium cepa:* the nasal discharge is bland and the tears are acrid.

Because onions also cause a pattern of symptoms which resembles hay fever and other respiratory allergies, *Allium cepa* is likewise an effective medicine for these allergies as long as the child's symptoms match.

ALLIUM CEPA

Allium cepa is often very effective in treating individual bouts of the common cold and respiratory allergies; however, it is not effective in curing a child's tendency to get recurrent colds or allergic reactions. Such a child needs to be prescribed a constitutional medicine by a professional homeopath. A deeper-acting medicine will help strengthen the body to significantly reduce the number of times the child gets ill.

Keynote Symptoms

- Profuse, acrid nasal discharge
- Profuse, bland tearing of the eyes
- Worse in a warm room; better in the open air

Modalities

Worse: warm rooms; getting wet; cold, damp winds.
Better: open air; cold room.

Primary Indicated Conditions

allergies   earache
colic   laryngitis
common cold

ANAS BARBARIAE,
HEPATITIS ET CORDIS/Anas barb
(Common name: Heart and liver of a duck)

Overview

Anas barb, which is popularly marketed as *Oscillococcinum* (Os-seel-lo-kok-si-num) is presently the most popular flu medicine in France, and it is becoming increasingly popular in the United States. It may not be easy to pronounce or spell, but it is wonderfully effective in treating influenza.

ANAS BARBARIAE, HEPATITIS ET CORDIS/Anas barb

Research published in the *British Journal of Clinical Pharmacology* (March, 1989) has proven its efficacy. This study of 487 flu patients showed that a significant number of patients who were given *Anas barb* recovered from the flu faster than those patients who were given a placebo.

Anas barb is made from the heart and liver of a duck. Although it may seem odd to some people that organs from a fowl could have therapeutic value, it is commonly acknowledged that chicken soup has beneficial therapeutic effects in fighting infection, a finding which scientific research has confirmed. Since chicken soup is made with chicken parts, perhaps *Anas barb* derives some of its infection-fighting properties from the duck's organs.

What gives chicken or duck organs these properties is still unknown. However, biologists and epidemiologists have observed that 80 percent of ducks carry every known influenza virus in their digestive tracts. Perhaps the microdoses of these viruses in *Anas barb* help the body treat the flu and prevent future bouts of it. Perhaps the homeopathic principle is again in evidence here.

Research and clinical experience has repeatedly shown that *Anas barb* is most effective in the 200th potency. Because of this, homeopathic manufacturers usually make available only this potency. Due to the exceedingly small amount of the substance used in this medicine, a single duck's internal organs can benefit thousands of ill people.

(*Anas barb* is manufactured as *Oscillococcinum* by the homeopathic company Boiron, Inc. This same ingredient is also manufactured by Dolisos under the name *Flu Solution* and is included in a combination medicine sold by Longevity Pure Medicines in a product called *Cold and Flu*.)

General Characteristics

Anas barb does not have widely confirmed individualizing symptoms. Some homeopaths consider it a generic influenza

ANAS BARBARIAE, HEPATITIS ET CORDIS/Anas barb

remedy. The common symptoms of the flu include a fever, body aches, general weakness, and a runny nose or cough.

It is most effective if taken within forty-eight hours of the onset of the flu. If you decide to try to use homeopathic medicines for your child's flu after that amount of time, you should probably try another homeopathic medicine.

Anas barb is also effective in treating the common cold, though it is not as consistently effective as it is in treating the flu.

Keynote Symptoms

- Symptoms of influenza or common cold during the first forty-eight hours

Primary Indicated Conditions

common cold   influenza

APIS MELLIFICA/Apis
(Common name: Crushed bee)

Overview

Bee venom creates a local symptom of burning, stinging pain and swelling. It could also cause a simple case of hives or more complicated syndromes of respiratory problems or digestive disorders, or even severe reactions such as anaphylactic shock—all symptoms and conditions which homeopathic doses of bee venom are known to prevent or cure.

Bee venom contains a protein that triggers a histamine reaction which can cause an allergic response. Because it causes symptoms of allergy, homeopathic doses of bee venom can also cure them. As you might predict, *Apis* is also useful for insect bites or bee stings in which there is much swelling, as well as burning, stinging pains.

APIS MELLIFICA/Apis

Folk wisdom has long acknowledged the value of bee venom in treating arthritis. Numerous people have reported that their arthritis disappeared shortly after getting stung by a bee. Because of this, some people have purposefully gotten a bee sting for relief. However, homeopaths assume that bee stings are only beneficial to those people who have arthritic symptoms that resemble a bee sting: swelling at the site of the pain, burning and stinging pain, reduction of pain from cold applications, and aggravation of pain from warm or hot applications. Homeopaths also suggest that it is considerably easier and less painful to take homeopathic doses of bee (*Apis*) than it is to get stung by one.

General Characteristics

One way you can tell if a child needs a homeopathic dose of bee is to examine a bee itself. Bees are violently reactive: they are easily irritated and will sting offenders or anyone threatening them. They are also restless, never staying on one flower too long. Similarly, children who need *Apis* are easily irritated and have quick tempers. They are restless and like to keep busy, even when ill.

A child who needs *Apis* has an inflammatory condition that creates great burning and hypersensitivity. He cannot stand the slightest touch of his inflamed part. He is fidgety and irritable, with a tendency to be clumsy. He drops things easily. He is hard to please, and like the bee who gives honey to the queen but is afraid that someone may steal the honey or the queen, he is easily jealous. He often experiences a physical illness shortly after a fit of jealousy or rage, or even after hearing bad news.

Children who need *Apis* also have symptoms similar to what bee venom causes: swelling, burning, and stinging pain, which is aggravated by heat and ameliorated by cold. Bee venom is known to cause swelling, both locally and throughout the whole body. Likewise, a child who will benefit from

APIS MELLIFICA/Apis

Apis will have swelling of individual parts (eyelids, lips, face, hands, feet, joints) as well as overall body swelling. The swelling is usually bright red and shiny and of a soft type in which the skin easily pits upon pressure. Also, like a bee sting, the affected part is very sensitive to touch.

It is difficult to know what type of pain infants experience. However, when they shriek with pain in a high pitch, it is likely that they are experiencing some type of stinging or pricking pain which may be relieved by a dose of *Apis*. These infants will be very irritable, will cry easily, and will be very sensitive to touch.

Apis is sometimes indicated for infants or children who develop symptoms after a vaccination. These symptoms may vary considerably, though the indications for giving *Apis* include the above-mentioned general characteristics.

Bee venom is also known to treat certain symptoms of allergy. Research published in the *British Journal of Clinical Pharmacology* showed that *Apis* inhibited the numbers of basophils, which are the white blood cells related to the allergic response of the body. *Apis* is one of the primary homeopathic medicines for treating hives, when there is puffiness of individual parts or a generalized swelling of the entire body. Like most of the symptoms that *Apis* is effective in treating, the hives are worse in heat or by warmth and are relieved by cold or cool applications.

A child who will benefit from *Apis* usually has a dry mouth, yet he is generally not thirsty, even though he may have an inflammatory condition or a fever. If he is thirsty, he wants milk, which seems soothing to him.

The symptoms are characteristically worse on the right side or, occasionally, begin on the right side and move to the left.

Keynote Symptoms

- Swelling
- Burning and stinging pain

APIS MELLIFICA/Apis

- Aggravation from heat and warm applications; amelioration from cold and cool applications

Modalities

Worse: warmth; warmth of a bed; touch; right side; pressure; late afternoon (especially at 3:00 P.M.).
Better: cold applications, cold bath, open air, uncovering, motion, sitting erect.

Primary Indicated Conditions

allergies	insect bites
chickenpox	measles
conjunctivitis	sore throat
hives	styes

ARNICA MONTANA/Arnica
(Common names: Arnica, Leopard's bane)

Overview

More people probably get introduced to (and become excited by) homeopathy through *Arnica* than any other homeopathic medicine. Whether it is given to children after they fall and hurt themselves, to a family member who has aches and pains after a day of physical labor, or to anyone for a sprain or strain, *Arnica* is a medicine *par excellence* for treating the common injury.

The Leopard's bane, from which *Arnica* is made, is a bright yellow, multipetaled flower that often grows on hillsides. This convenient location is wonderfully practical for people who fall when climbing mountains. In folk medicine it was called *fall herb*, because it was commonly used as a poultice by mountain dwellers who fell and injured themselves.

ARNICA MONTANA/Arnica

Taken internally, however, arnica is a poisonous herb which directly affects the heart and its blood vessels. It causes overcontraction of the heart and ultimately an enlarged heart. In lesser, though still harmful, doses it causes blood vessel dilation, then stasis (stagnation), and finally increased swelling, leading to black and blue bruising and a general bruised feeling. Although these symptoms may sound intimidating, homeopathically *Arnica* is used in such a small dose that toxic reactions are not possible.

Orthopedic surgeon Robert Becker strongly affirmed his success in using *Arnica* in his book, *Cross Currents,* stating, "In many years of orthopedic practice, I have treated hundreds of sprained ankles. Provided that the ligament is not completely torn, I have found that simply rubbing on *Arnica* ointment within a few hours of the injury results in practically instantaneous and complete relief of pain, a rapid and complete resolution of swelling, and a rapid (one to two days) disappearance of the blood clot. I know of no other agent, FDA approved or otherwise, that can match the efficiency of *Arnica* in this respect."

Because of its many uses in first aid and in emergencies, *Arnica* should have a prominent place in your home medicine cabinet.

General Characteristics

Arnica is the primary homeopathic medicine for treating injury. It is the best medicine for the initial shock and trauma of injury, and due to its ability to significantly reduce pain, it is considered the aspirin of homeopathy for injuries. As a result of its affinity to the heart and its blood vessels, *Arnica* is extremely effective in regulating heart activity after injury and in stopping hemorrhage, both externally and internally. *Arnica* also helps the body to absorb blood clots lodged in the tissues.

Arnica helps repair damaged blood vessels from bruises. It

ARNICA MONTANA/Arnica

will stimulate healing by helping the body reabsorb blood from injuries and reduce pain and swelling. *Arnica* is also effective for ruptures of the tiny blood vessels in the eye which cause the sclera (the whites of the eye) to become red. It also helps to resolve the pooling of blood under the skin, as in a black eye or a bruise.

A common symptom of shock from injury is nonrecognition of the seriousness of the problem. Typically, someone in shock thinks he is OK. He may walk a short distance away from the accident saying "Nothing's wrong," but then may collapse. Because shock causes reduced blood flow to the brain, a person in shock is not thinking clearly. It is thus recommended to treat an injured child for shock whether they seem seriously hurt or not. The primary symptoms of a child in shock are a cold, pale or gray face, general weakness, rapid or weak heart rate, reduced alertness, confusion or unconsciousness, and shallow, irregular breathing. *Arnica* should be an integral part of treatment for shock, along with general first-aid measures and, when appropriate, professional medical care.

Because of the value of *Arnica* in dealing with shock, reducing pain and swelling, and helping the body reabsorb blood, it is the most common remedy given to a child before and after surgery. Many homeopaths almost routinely give it to mothers and newborn infants because of the shock and trauma commonly experienced during childbirth. It is also beneficial for baby boys who get circumcised.

Arnica is an effective medicine for head injuries, even head injuries that may have occurred years before. It may also be good for various types of old injuries which are still bothersome. The exceptions to this general application are old nerve injuries, for which *Hypericum* is indicated, and old knee injuries, for which *Ruta* is helpful.

Arnica is the best medicine for a bruised feeling from an injury. If, for instance, you touch a spot on a child and it feels sore or bruised to them, *Arnica* should be given.

ARNICA MONTANA/Arnica

In addition to being helpful in treating muscle aches after overexertion, *Arnica* is invaluable as a preventive medicine when taken either before or after a workout. Taking *Arnica* will prevent the stiffness that often occurs the next morning. *Arnica* is also the first medicine to consider for treating dislocated joints.

A common indicaton for the use of *Arnica* is when a child feels restless in bed, not because she is actually restless but because she feels the bed is too hard. Such a child may have a bruised feeling all over and feel exhausted. The stiffness from overexertion creates a tenderness in the muscle tissue which *Arnica* can relieve.

For muscle aches, sprains, and strains, give *Arnica* tablets internally *and* also apply it externally as a gel, lotion, ointment, or spray. A child who receives a head injury need only take potentized internal doses of *Arnica*.

Note that external applications of *Arnica* are not recommended when the skin is broken. External applications of *Arnica* can cause irritation when applied to open wounds. *Calendula* or *Hypericum* is indicated for cuts and wounds.

Keynote Symptoms

- Shock and trauma of injury
- Bruising and hemorrhaging from injury
- Muscle aches from overexertion
- Pre- and post-surgery
- Head injuries
- Old injuries which are still bothersome

Modalities

Worse: overexertion; cold; hot; motion; touch; jar; hard bed.
Better: lying down; open air.

ARNICA MONTANA/Arnica

Primary Indicated Conditions

backache

birth trauma

bleeding

bruises

circumcision

eye injuries

fracture

head injuries

jet lag

muscle injuries

shock from injury

smashed fingers or toes

sprains and strains

surgery

toothache

ARSENICUM ALBUM/Arsenicum
(Common name: White arsenic)

Overview

Arsenic is a deadly poison which creates burning in the mouth, constriction of the throat, and gastric pain. Ingesting it can cause violent vomiting and diarrhea, both of which may contain blood. It also leads to diminished or suppressed urine, muscle cramps, headache, and great weakness. Ultimately, it can cause significant dehydration and cramps with collapse, leading to death in only six hours after ingestion.

It is such an effective and often unsuspected poison that the early 1800s are sometimes called the "Age of Arsenic" because of its popularity during that time as a means of assassination in Europe.

People, however, can develop a tolerance to arsenic when they are given continuous, small doses of it. In the Far East there are still arsenic eaters, people who ingest normally fatal doses but who have developed a tolerance to the poison. Animals can also tolerate small doses of arsenic and even benefit from it. Horses are given small doses to give them especially sleek and glossy coats. It is given to turkeys to aid breeding and to prevent disease.

ARSENICUM ALBUM/Arsenicum

Arsenic was used in conventional medicine in the nineteenth century, usually for ulcers, skin diseases, and certain fevers. More recently, various preparations of arsenic have been used in the manufacture of dyes and pesticides.

Arsenic also has the peculiar attribute of being impossible to destroy, even by fire. It can combine with many other substances to create a wide variety of compounds, but the element itself remains immutable.

Although arsenic can be toxic when ingested in crude doses, homeopathic doses in *Arsenicum* are so small that they are widely recognized as safe.

General Characteristics

The most typical characteristic of a child who needs *Arsenicum* is the onset of symptoms at or after midnight. The child awakens suddenly with a fever, headache, breathing difficulty, or digestive problem.

Burning pains and burning discharges are most typical. There is burning in the head, throat, stomach, bladder, or vagina. There may be burning discharges from the eyes, nose, or vagina and a burning sensation on urinating or passing stools. Despite this burning, the pains are relieved by heat and warm applications.

Even though these children may experience burning symptoms, they are in general very chilly. They may even feel like there is ice in their veins. Sometimes a common cold, sinusitis, cough, or allergy may begin after a child is chilled.

The child will have a very dry mouth and great thirst, but for frequent sips rather than gulps of water. He is often worse from cold food and drinks, especially milk and ice cream, and from wheat, sugar, and coffee. He is also worse from overeating melon, strawberries, and other fruits. He is relieved by warm food and drinks.

Arsenicum has been called "the horse's remedy" because

ARSENICUM ALBUM/Arsenicum

people who need it are like horses: they have power and endurance but are very restless, high-strung, and easily prone to fright.

Children who need *Arsenicum* tend to be very anxious, whether it is about something specific or just a generalized anxious feeling. This anxiety displays itself in physical and mental restlessness. The child feels compelled to move from bed to chair, chair to bed, and room to room. He is fearful, and anticipates his troubles worsening. He thinks that his problem is much more serious than it is. He may repeatedly ask his parents what is wrong with him. He is more fastidious than usual, and this anxious and fussy meticulousness will compel him to clean his room, even though he may feel quite ill. (Parents usually realize that this behavior suggests something is definitely wrong!)

Despite his restlessness, the child who will benefit from *Arsenicum* feels great fatigue and exhaustion. He may become weakened from the slightest exertion. This weakness seems to be out of proportion with the child's problem. Parents often assume that their child is feigning illness. Sometimes, his symptoms of exhaustion may begin after completing a major achievement.

He likes getting attention from others, and he may even perk up from his ill and exhausted state in order to get it. He feels greater anxiety when alone and desires company, though he is quite demanding on others. He expects others to be at his beck and call. He feels relief from talking, especially about his problems. He is easily frightened, and is particularly scared of being alone and being in the dark. His vivid imagination conjures up creative fears, and his restlessness takes him out of his own bed and into his parents'.

He is also anxious about his health and about food. Because he thinks that he is much more ill than he is, he encourages his parents to take him to doctor after doctor to try to prove it. The perfectionism for which these kind of teenagers are known may show itself in a sense that they can never be too thin. These teenagers sometimes have an aversion to all food, or become anorexic because they have a fixed idea or a delusion that they are fat.

This kind of child is also very fussy. He is very particular about what foods he likes and doesn't like, what games he wants to play, what places he likes; in fact, he tends to have strong opinions about most subjects. He has fixed ideas about what is the right or best way of understanding and doing things and he is usually intolerant of others' perceptions and methods.

Most commonly, children who will benefit from *Arsenicum* are sensitive to noise which distracts them and to odors such as smoke, gas, or perfume. They also tend to experience more symptoms on the right side of their body.

Keynote Symptoms

- Physical and mental restlessness
- Anxiety that the condition will worsen
- Burning pains and discharges
- Very chilly
- Great thirst, but for only sips at a time
- Symptoms worse at and after midnight

Modalities

Worse: at and after midnight; cold; cold food or drinks; being alone; a watery fruit and vegetable diet; milk; wheat; sugar; ice cream; alcohol; coffee.

Better: warm temperature or applications; warm foods or drinks; better from talking, especially about his problems; being in company; motion.

ARSENICUM ALBUM/Arsenicum

Primary Indicated Conditions

allergies	headaches
anxiety	impetigo
asthma	indigestion
common cold	influenza
conjunctivitis	insomnia
diarrhea	nervous restlessness
fever	sinusitis
food poisoning	sore throat

BELLADONNA
(Common name: Deadly nightshade)

Overview

The word *belladonna* is derived from two Italian words: *bella* "beautiful" and *donna* "woman." In ancient times large pupils were associated with beauty; *Belladonna* received its name because it has the ability to dilate the pupils of the eyes.

This pupil dilation is caused by one of the primary ingredients in belladonna, atropine. Eye doctors are better able to look into the eye after administering this substance. Because belladonna creates dilated pupils in non-homeopathic doses, it also has the ability to heal a person who has this symptom as a part of his illness. This characteristic symptom helps homeopaths prescribe this medicine for infants who are not able to describe their symptoms.

A known hallucinogen, belladonna is so powerful that people who place some of its leaves or flowers under their pillow during sleep tend to experience vivid dreams. Because of this, *Belladonna* is a very common homeopathic medicine for a child who tends to have an active dream life, especially when ill.

Belladonna contains numerous powerful chemicals called

BELLADONNA

alkaloids, including atropine, hyoscyamine, and scopolamine. These alkaloids affect the nervous system, specifically the autonomic system (the autonomic nervous system controls various functions of the body, including digestion, blood circulation, and reproductive activities). It causes stimulation of the sympathetic nerves and inhibition of the parasympathetic nerves, causing paralysis of certain muscle groups and the drying up of various bodily secretions, including saliva, mucus, perspiration, and digestive juices.

Although belladonna is a known poisonous plant, even conventional physicians acknowledge its therapeutic powers. It is one of the primary ingredients in the common over-the-counter cold product Dristan. The standard pharmacological text, Goodman and Gilman's *Basis in Pharmacology,* relates that normal medical doses of atropine block the parasympathetic nerves, resulting in the drying up of mucous membranes, and yet, it also recognizes that exceedingly small doses of atropine have the opposite effect: it causes increased secretion of mucus. This medically recognized dual effect of atropine provides additional evidence of the homeopathic action of medicines, since most physicians incorrectly assume that drugs primarily have a single effect which is simply amplified or diminished depending upon the dose.

General Characteristics

You can often deduce that *Belladonna* is the correct medicine for your child simply by looking at her appearance. Her face is often flushed red, as are her lips, tongue, gums, and if the inner ear is inflamed, the outer ear is also red. Her eyes are glassy and the pupils are dilated.

A fever commonly accompanies the condition. It is usually very high with a radiating heat: you can sometimes feel the heat emanating from your child's skin. Characteristically, she has an extremely hot head but cold extremities. Along with the heat, she has a dry mouth, tongue, throat, and nose. Her

BELLADONNA

skin is also dry, though she may sweat on her covered parts. Despite this heat and dryness, she is not usually thirsty. If she is thirsty, it may be for lemons or lemonade.

A child who needs *Belladonna* usually has a sudden onset and sudden disappearance of pain, whether it is a headache, cramp, twitching, or toothache. The pain is typically intense and of a throbbing, stitching, or stabbing nature. The child may actually feel her own full and bounding pulse.

Headaches accompany many conditions that this kind of child experiences. The headaches are often throbbing and are aggravated by touch, motion, and while lying flat. Some relief is experienced by sitting up or by gradually applying pressure to the painful areas.

Along with their intense pains, children who need *Belladonna* are restless, distraught, delirious, and may groan, and even bite or pull the hair of people close by. These children may suffer from delusional states and hallucinations, especially during high fevers. Most typically, they see monsters in the dark, and upon closing their eyes, they are apt to have active, often frightful visions of people, animals, or simply lights and colors.

Michael Carlston, M.D., a homeopath in Santa Rosa, California, used *Belladonna* for a child who had recurrent ear infections along with various behavioral problems. This child had many fears and was easily startled. He was scared of the stuffed bunny in the doctor's office, and he didn't like going to birthday parties because a child would sometimes accidentally pop a balloon, which would seriously startle him. When Dr. Carlston also learned that this little boy had a strong tendency to bite (he even bit his six-month-old brother), *Belladonna* was prescribed. After taking it, not only did the child no longer experience earaches, he now plays with the doctor's stuffed bunny and, like most children, he loves birthday parties. Such is the power of homeopathic medicines to treat both infections and behavior problems.

Belladonna is an extremely common remedy for the child

BELLADONNA

who has difficulty sleeping when ill. Her sleep is restless, and she may jerk during sleep. She tends to have wild dreams. She may even see ghosts or imagine frightening things. She may scream out in her sleep, not just because of pain but because she is frightened. Other symptoms that the child experiences are sensitivity to touch, light, and noise. The child prefers to be in the dark, quiet, and comfortably propped up in bed.

Prescribing note: Belladonna is a fast-acting medicine. If it is the correct remedy, you will usually notice distinct improvement within a couple of hours. (And improvement is usually noticed within fifteen minutes.)

Keynote Symptoms

- Sudden onset and disappearance of symptoms, especially fevers, spasms, cramps, twitchings
- Dry, hot, reddened face and mucous membranes
- Throbbing, stitching, and stabbing pains
- Hypersensitive to touch, jar, or light

Modalities

Worse: cold air; more symptoms on right side; motion; noise; being jarred or touched; 3:00 P.M.; at night, especially after midnight; stooping or bending; lying down; looking at bright lights.
Better: warm room; being at rest; standing or sitting erect.

Primary Indicated Conditions

bedwetting	conjunctivitis
boils	cough
chickenpox	earache
colic	fever
common cold	headaches

BELLADONNA

heatstroke   sinusitis
hepatitis   sore throat
influenza   teething
measles   toothache
mumps

BRYONIA ALBA/Bryonia
(Common name: Wild hops)
Overview

The name *Bryonia* is derived from the Greek word *bryo*, which means "I shoot, or sprout." This refers to the vigorous and active stages of this plant's growth. It is a vine-like plant that covers trees and shrubs. The stems are rough to the touch and have short, prickly hairs.

Children who will benefit from *Bryonia* are similarly prickly, both psychologically and physiologically. They tend to be irritable and prefer to be left alone and unbothered. They have many sharp, tearing, and even stabbing pains, and dry, rough, hacking coughs. Yet, quite distinct from the active growth of *Bryonia,* children who need this medicine are made considerably worse by any motion.

General Characteristics

Bryonia is the grumpy bear medicine: the child wants to be left alone and is irritable if disturbed. He doesn't want company and will grumble, snarl, and snap if necessary to keep others away. He resents intrusions and doesn't want other people to bother him.

The child has an uneasy feeling that compels him to move, but he feels worse when he does. He becomes increasingly irritable as his ailment progresses. He is so sensitive to motion that his symptoms are aggravated even by talking (movement of the jaw), swallowing (movement of the throat), and coughing (movement of the chest), and even thinking (moving from

BRYONIA ALBA/Bryonia

one thought to another). His head hurts when he moves his eyes or when he bends down.

One of the ways that this type of child deals with his hypersensitivity is by trying to remain perfectly still. He also tries to inhibit motion by holding his chest when he coughs or holding his throat when he talks. He will lie on whatever part of his body feels painful because he feels better from applying firm pressure, though he cringes from the lightest touch.

A child who needs *Bryonia* will be aggravated by the passive motion of being carried or lifted. He will also tend to be peevish, asking for something and then refusing it once it is offered. He has a peevish appetite, too: he will want, even demand, food, but he doesn't know what kind of food he wants.

Typically, children who need *Bryonia* will feel less well after eating. Their symptoms tend to be aggravated by eating beans, bread, cabbage, fruit, milk, fatty foods, and vegetables.

They tend to be sensitive to light, so they prefer to sit in the dark.

Bryonia is most often helpful for children living in damp climates. It is commonly given to a child who becomes ill after getting chilled or after having a cold drink when he is warm. The ailment may also begin after the child has a fit of anger or embarrassment.

Quite distinct from children helped by *Aconitum* or *Belladonna,* who have a sudden onset of symptoms, the child who needs *Bryonia* tends to have a slow onset of symptoms. He may, at first, have a simple cold, which may develop into a headache, cough, or fever in the next couple of days.

Dryness is another of the distinct symptoms. The mouth and lips will be dry, and the tongue is dry and coated, usually white. The throat and larynx are dry and raw. The digestive juices are minimal as well. Food lies undigested in the stomach and feels like a heavy lump or a stone. The child is habitually constipated, with dry, hard, large stools. His cough is usually dry too. Along with this dryness is great thirst, usually for cold drinks.

BRYONIA ALBA/Bryonia

Cool and open air is beneficial to those children who need *Bryonia*. A child in great discomfort will be noticeably relieved when a window is opened. The coolness not only benefits him physically, but mentally too. In addition to disliking warm rooms, these children sometimes cannot stand the heat of the sun either.

The pains of children who will benefit from *Bryonia* will usually be stitching, stabbing, or congestive. Their chest or abdominal pains will be sharp, aggravated by any motion or the lightest touch, and will be lessened by firm pressure.

Most often, the symptoms are worse on the right side of the body.

Despite being ill, the child who needs *Bryonia* tends to think, worry, and even dream about his responsibilities, whether they be at work, school, or around the house.

Keynote Symptoms

- Symptoms made worse by any motion

- Sharp, stitching pains

- Dryness of mucous membranes, especially the mouth and rectum

- Relief of symptoms by applying pressure to painful parts

- Aggravated in warm rooms; prefers to have a window open

- Thirsty for cold drinks

- Desire to be alone; irritable

Modalities

Worse: motion; being jarred; warmth; warm rooms; heat of the sun; during summer; after eating cabbage, beans, bread,

BRYONIA ALBA/Bryonia

fruits; swallowing; sneezing; laying on painless side; stooping; moving the eyes.

Better: lying completely still; cool, open air; cold water; cold food; lying on painful side; pressure on painful parts; dark room.

Primary Indicated Conditions

anger	headaches
backache	indigestion
colic	influenza
common cold	measles
constipation	pneumonia
cough	sprains and strains
fracture	

CALCAREA CARBONICA/Calcarea carb
(Common name: Calcium carbonate)

Overview

Calcium is one of the most abundant minerals on our planet, and it is likewise one of the primary minerals of the human body. Approximately 99 percent of calcium assimilated by the body goes to the teeth and bones, with the remaining 1 percent of calcium used for several vital bodily functons: muscle growth and contraction, blood clotting, and enzyme activation. Despite its importance to the human body, calcium is not easily absorbed by it. Numerous foods and drinks can inhibit calcium assimilation, including alcohol, fats, caffeine, bran, excessive protein, and oxalic acid-rich foods (chard, spinach, rhubard, and chocolate), and phosphorus-rich foods and drinks (junk food and soda drinks are the worst offenders).

A basic aspect of homeopathic theory is that a homeopathic medicine made from a specific nutrient will help the body absorb that nutrient more efficiently. Because calcium is so important to the growing fetus, infant, and child, it is no wonder that *Calcarea carbonica* is a vital medicine for infants and children.

Homeopathic manufacturers obtain their calcium carbonate from the inner layer of an oyster shell. Living on the bottom of an ocean bed, oysters have only one range of motion: they open and close their shells with vice-like strength. Passive and sedentary, the oyster, like the child helped by *Calcarea carbonica,* is content with simply being and passively sitting. These children stubbornly avoid exertion, and if they must move, they do so slowly.

General Characteristics

Calcarea carbonica is most often given to the infant or child who is fat or who at least has flabby skin tone. She tends to be very stubborn, especially when she is tired or if she is forced to do anything. She is mentally and physically slow, and usually starts walking and talking at a later age than other children. She also avoids any mental or physical effort, not because she is lazy, but because she becomes easily exhausted and because she hates being laughed at by others for doing things slowly or improperly. She is sensitive to being teased or criticized.

Along with her slowness is a sense of complacency. She is content wherever she is. This complacency is part of the reason that she is slow, sometimes very slow, in learning to walk. She also likes to play alone or do little or nothing for long periods of time, not being aware of what is going on around her. She tends to sit in a slumped posture.

Despite her slowness, the child can be bright, though she may not be performing up to her capabilities. Part of her character is that she prefers to do things at her own pace and doesn't like to be hurried.

CALCAREA CARBONICA/Calcarea carb

She has many fears and, as a result, she tends to be very clingy. She is afraid of the dark, and of insects, animals, and heights. She is afraid of new challenges and strongly prefers her own routine. She also is afraid that something may happen to her, and a fear that everybody is looking at her in suspicion. She tends to have terrifying dreams.

This type of child sweats profusely on her head and feet, especially at night and from the slightest exertion. She is very chilly, though she will have warm, even burning feet in bed at night. The child is often affected by cold weather, tending to get recurrent infections during the winter months, including colds, coughs, ear infections, and sore throats. In contrast, infants who need *Calcarea carbonica* will not be as noticeably chilly and in fact may be warm, except the feet, which will be very cold. Whether the child is warm or not, she will be aggravated by exposure to cold.

These kinds of children crave eggs (especially soft-boiled eggs), carbohydrates (breads, pasta, potatoes), ice cream, sweets, and salt. They crave cold drinks (the colder, the better). They sometimes also crave indigestible items such as dirt, chalk, and coal. They are usually averse to hot foods, slimy foods, and mixed foods such as casseroles. They also dislike milk and may even have a milk allergy, experiencing indigestion or various other symptoms after drinking it.

Most typically, these infants and children have large, round heads, distended abdomens, chronically swollen neck glands, and recurrent runny noses. They have sour discharges and odors. The breath, vomit, stools, and perspiration usually smell sour. The child may have diarrhea, though it will alternate with constipation. Oddly enough, the child feels better when she is constipated.

Prescribing note: Calcarea carbonica is more often prescribed based on its general characteristics than upon the specific local symptoms.

CALCAREA CARBONICA/Calcarea carb

Keynote Symptoms

- fat or flabby and fair-skinned
- chilly and easily tired
- perspiration on the head and feet
- sour sweat, smell, and stools
- stubborn

Modalities

Worse: cold; change of weather from warm to cold; exposure to cold water; after any exertion, physical or mental; after midnight.

Better: warmth; dry weather; when constipated; lying on the painful side.

Primary Indicated Conditions

canker sores	diarrhea
colic	earache
common cold	indigestion
constipation	teething
diaper rash	

CALENDULA
(Common name: Marigold)

Overview

Marigold flowers are said to bloom on the calends (the first day of the month, according to the ancient Julian calendar), and it is from this that they got their Latin name.

CALENDULA

Calendula is more often used in homeopathy as an external appliation than as an internal medicine. It is commonly sold as a tincture, a gel, a spray, a cream, an oil, and even as a soap. See the section "External Applications" in part 5.

General Characteristics

Calendula is a homeopathic antiseptic, in part because of its organic iodine content. It helps a wound resist infection and aids in the healing of wounds and burns by promoting granulation of tissues. When externally applied, it prevents pus formation and is soothing and nourishing to the skin. *Calendula* also promotes degranulation of scars, helping to break them down to create new, healthy tissue. The yellow and orange colors of the marigold flower are derived from carotenoids and flavonoids, which have beneficial and regenerative effects on the skin.

Calendula is also composed of more than thirty chemical compounds, including salicylic acid, which is the primary active ingredient in aspirin. This ingredient explains why it has some pain-reducing action.

Its nutritious nature soothes the pain of canker sores and reduces redness and inflammation in the eyes, while its adhesive nature coats the inflamed area and provides relief.

Prescribing note: Calendula should not be used externally on deep wounds because it tends to quickly heal the external part, leaving the deeper part open and subject to abscess formation.

Keynote Symptoms

- Cuts and wounds from injury and surgery
- First-degree burns
- Hemorrhages from an injury

CALENDULA

Primary Indicated Conditions

bleeding	cuts and abrasions
burns	diaper rash
canker sores	eye injuries
conjunctivitis	scars

CANTHARIS
(Common name: Spanish fly)

Overview

Spanish fly is commonly thought to be an aphrodisiac, but actually, it is such an irritant to the genitals and the urinary system that any person who ingests it wishes to rub or touch the genitals unceasingly.

Dried Spanish fly, also called blister beetle, contains uric, formic, and acetic acid. As a means of self-defense when alive, this beetle's skin will cause blistering if it is simply touched. If taken internally, Spanish fly has a special affinity for causing symptoms of the urinary tract, the lower bowel, and the skin.

E. B. Nash, M.D., one of the great homeopaths in the nineteenth century, said, "If I were to select the one remedy with which to prove the truth of the formula, *Similia similibus curentur* (the law of similars), I think this would be the one." Constantine Hering, M.D., the father of American homeopathy, was so confident of the value of *Cantharis* in treating burns that he would challenge skeptics to burn their fingers, and then cure them by putting their fingers in water which contained *Cantharis*.

General Characteristics

When a child has a burning sensation on urinating, the first medicine to consider is *Cantharis*. There is usually a great urgency and a constant desire to urinate, yet she is able to urinate only a couple of drops at a time and experiences burning and cutting pain before, during, or after urination. These pains make the child very restless. Typically, the child experiences a sudden onset of these symptoms.

Although *Cantharis* is known to cure extremely painful burning urination, it is also effective for even mildly burning urinaton. It can cure burning pains in various places, including the brain, eyes, throat, chest, stomach, the whole intestinal tract, and the ovaries. The child may feel as though she is on fire. Despite these internal burning pains, she may feel chilly externally.

The child tends to be thirsty but will not want to drink. Occasionally, she will have throat symptoms. It hurts to swallow, and it hurts even more to urinate. The throat, like the bladder, has spasms and has great difficulty letting anything in or out. The throat and the bladder are also very sensitive to touch. The child will be averse to food as well.

If she has any discharge from the mouth, throat, chest, or urinary tract, it will be of a ropy, tenacious consistency.

Children who need *Cantharis* are, in general, hypersensitive, as evidenced by a mental state that is irritated by the slightest touch. They are also restless and want to change positions frequently. The child may be in a mental frenzy: possessed by strange ideas, turbulent emotions, delirium, and even sexual fantasies. There may be such strong emotional and mental activity that it disturbs the child's sleep at night.

Keynote Symptoms

- Burning pains

- Pains before, during, and after urination

- Painful urination of only drops at a time

- Restlessness

CANTHARIS

Modalities

Worse: before, during, or after urination; motion or touch; drinking fluids, especially coffee.
Better: warmth; belching or passing gas; at night; cold applications.

Primary Indicated Conditions

bladder infection   burns

CHAMOMILLA
(Common name: Chamomile)

Overview

One of the very early homeopaths, Dr. Charles Hempel, called *Chamomilla* the "catnip of homeopathy" because of its soothing effect, especially on children. It is such a powerfully calming medicine that homeopaths use it to treat the most irritable stages of infancy and childhood.

The herb chamomile is so common that some people consider it a weed. It grows in small strips of land and even in cracks in the sidewalk. Whereas most plants would be stifled or die from the trampling that chamomile gets, it actually thrives on it. An old poem highlights this unusual ability of chamomile:

"like a chamomile bed—
the more it is trodden
the more it will spread."

Quite distinct from other weeds which take over an area and make it difficult for other plants to grow, drooping or sickly plants tend to become invigorated when chamomile

CHAMOMILLA

grows near them. Because of these beneficial effects, chamomile is sometimes called the "plant's physician."

The child who needs *Chamomilla* is in some ways like the flower. While the flower irrepressibly grows wherever and whenever it can, the child who it will help is irrepressibly irritable. Like the flower that thrives on being trampled, this child's irritability is inflamed by any attention he gets. Nothing provides relief; the only exception is rocking or carrying the child.

Chamomile is a member of the daisy family, the Composites, as are other homeopathic medicines such as *Arnica*, *Cina*, and *Millefolium*.

General Characteristics

A child who needs *Chamomilla* may normally be nice and sweet when he is well, but this Dr. Jekyll turns into a Mr. Hyde during an illness. *Chamomilla* is one of the leading medicines for children who are angry. The child cannot bear it—the pain, other people, himself, or anything; he cannot even bear to be looked at or spoken to. He demands things but then discards the things for which he has asked. The only way to provide relief, albeit temporary relief, is to rock or carry the child. This hyperrestless child may be relieved briefly by the passive soothing motion, but shortly after putting him down again the screaming and crying returns.

The typical image of a temper tantrum resembles the character of *Chamomilla*. The child is very tempermental; he snarls, throws things, is impatient, and whines. He may even bang his head against a wall. Various symptoms may arise after this emotional outburst, though it is as likely that physical symptoms will begin first which then lead to hyperirritability.

If an irritable child is punished and then has convulsions after his disciplining, *Chamomilla* should be seriously considered. It is also indicated when a nursing infant becomes sick shortly after the mother experiences hyperirritability.

CHAMOMILLA

In addition to being emotionally sensitive, these children are physically sensitive to light, noise, smell, taste, and touch. They are aggravated by heat, warm rooms, and warm applications, as well as by wind and open air. They do not want to be touched, except when rocked or carried.

Due to the child's irritability and his hypersensitivity to light and noise, he has great difficulty in sleeping, even when he is sleepy. Waking or sleeping, he tends to throw off whatever covers there are. His rage and irritability usually keep you awake too.

Chamomilla is also an effective medicine for treating pain, especially pain that seems out of proportion to the illness.

The appearance of the *Chamomilla* child will often signal its prescription. The child will look inflamed. One cheek may be red and hot, while the other is cold and pale. The head is warm and moist with sweat, and his feet will be hot and cannot endure being under the covers. He is usually aggravated by heat.

Not only does the child have a sour disposition but also sour-smelling stools, body odor, and gas.

He avoids warm drinks and is thirsty for cold drinks, especially for acidic drinks (such as lemonade or orange juice).

Although the child can go through his physical and psychological hell at any time, the worst times tend to be at 9:00 A.M. and 9:00 P.M.

Prescribing note: Some parents routinely give *Chamomilla* to their teething infant without adequately individualizing the infant's symptoms. Remember, there are other homeopathic remedies for teething in addition to *Chamomilla*.

Parents also sometimes get such good results with *Chamomilla* that they give it to their child for any slight pain, discomfort, or emotional upset. This routine prescribing can create its own problems because the child may then experience a proving of *Chamomilla*, that is, the frequent dosing of this remedy may create the irritability and anger that the infrequent dosing tends to cure.

CHAMOMILLA

Keynote Symptoms

- Very irritable
- Nothing pleases them, except being carried
- Hypersensitive, physically and psychologically
- Sour stools, vomit, sweat, and taste in the mouth
- Experiences pain out of proportion to the illness

Modalities

Worse: during teething; touch; at 9:00 A.M. or 9:00 P.M.; heat; wind; coffee.
Better: being carried or being driven in a car.

Primary Indicated Conditions

anger	indigestion
asthma	insomnia
colic	nervous restlessness
diarrhea	teething
earache	toothache

~

COLOCYNTHIS
(Common names: Bitter cucumber, Bitter apple)

Overview

Bitter cucumber belongs to the *Cucurbitaceae* family, the same family to which *Bryonia* belongs. It is a trailing plant which does not make firm attachments, as does *Bryonia*, but twists around other objects. Similarly, the bitter cucumber in excessive dosage causes cramping, gripping pains that make a person twist and writhe in pain.

COLOCYNTHIS

Its bristly stem and prickly leaves suggest an irritable, un-sociable nature; homeopathic doses of *Colocynthis* can offer relief to this type of child.

Colocynthis has an acute irritant effect on the gastro-intestinal system, provoking nausea, vomiting, and severe cramping. It also has an affinity for the nervous system, creating spasms and nerve pains.

General Characteristics

Children needing *Colocynthis* are primarily characterized by cramping pains and extreme irritability. Sometimes the physical pain triggers the psychological state, and other times it's vice versa. The severity of the pain, usually a cramping or shooting pain like an electric shock, causes the child to double up, which provides her some relief. She also feels some relief from firmly pressing a hard object or her fist into the source of the pain. She may lean over a chair, a bed, or a table in order to apply firm pressure to her pain. She may also lay on her belly as a way of applying pressure.

The pain usually consists of abdominal or uterine cramping, often accompanied by vomiting and diarrhea. It typically moves in waves, coming and going rapidly. It is usually worse on the left side, though right-sided pains are also sometimes felt.

Firm pressure may provide some relief at first, but later the abdomen will be sensitive and aggravated by any touch. Relief is felt with warm applications, though the relief is only temporary. Passing gas or a stool may ameliorate the symptoms.

The child is restless. The pain is so severe that she can't stay still. The symptoms are made worse by rest. Despite her restlessness, the pains are relieved by drinking caffeinated sodas.

The pain that the child feels is written on her face, which is dark red and may be distorted with pain. Preceding or concurrent with this pain is extreme irritability, frustration, and

COLOCYNTHIS

anger from the slightest cause. Grief may also precede the physical pain.

She is usually chilly and sensitive to cold, especially cold and damp weather. She may be extremely thirsty, though if she is nauseated she will vomit after any food or drink. She is particularly prone to vomiting after eating fruit or cheese. She tends to have a bitter taste in her mouth.

Keynote Symptoms

- Cramping, gripping pains
- Relief from bending double
- Relief from firm pressure
- Extreme irritability
- Illness comes after grief or anger

Modalities

Worse: after experiencing anger, grief, anguish, or embarrassment; eating or drinking (even small amounts); fruit, cheese; cold wind; damp cold weather; at 4:00 P.M.

Better: bending double; firm pressure; warm applications; passing gas or a stool; caffeinated sodas, coffee, tobacco.

Primary Indicated Conditions

anger   diarrhea
colic

EUPHRASIA
(Common name: Eyebright)

Overview

The name *Euphrasia* has Greek origins, derived from *Euphrasyne,* which means "gladness." *Euphrasyne* was one of the three Graces, and she was identified with joy and mirth. Because the herb was found to be such an effective medicine for the eyes, it was considered to bring gladness and joy to those who used it.

British poet John Milton mentioned *Euphrasia* when he wrote of how the Archangel Michael ministered to Adam after the fall:

> ". . . to nobler sights
> Michael from Adam's eyes the film removed,
> Then purged with ephrasine and rue
> His visual orbs, for he had much to see."

Some folklore about the origins of this herb's usage suggests that the *Doctrine of Signatures* may have alerted herbalists to its value. (The *Doctrine of Signatures* is an ancient theory that assumes that what an herb looks like and how it grows provides insight into its therapeutic value. This principle is thought to be a precursor to homeopathy and its law of similars.) As one writer said, "the purple and yellow spots and stripes which are upon the flowers of the Eyebright doth very much resemble the diseases of the eyes, as bloodshot, etc. by which signature it hath been found out that this herb is effectual for the curing of the same."

The medicine is prepared during the plant's flowering stages, which may be a factor in its value in treating people who suffer from hypersensitivity to flowers in bloom—the condition commonly called hay fever.

It has its greatest effect upon the mucous membranes, especially the eyes, eyelids, and the upper respiratory tract.

General Characteristics

Euphrasia is known for its beneficial action on children whose eyes water profusely and frequently, especially from an allergy.

EUPHRASIA

The tears burn the eyes and even irritate and redden the cheeks. The eyes feel as though pepper had been put in them. The margins of the lids are red, swollen, and burning. The frequent itching and burning of the eyes cause the child to blink often and to scratch and rub them.

The child may experience photophobia, a sensitivity to light. The eyes may exude a discharge at night, gluing the lids together upon waking.

Concurrently, there is often fluent, bland (nonirritating) nasal discharge. The nasal discharge is worse in the morning and may be accompanied by a cough and abundant expectoration. The nasal discharge may also be worse when the child is outside.

A headache may be present with the eye symptoms. The child also becomes chilly and has difficulty getting warm in bed. He may also have a tendency toward frequent yawning when walking in the open air.

Keynote Symptoms

- Profuse, acrid tearing
- Fluent, bland nasal discharge

Modalities

Worse: cold air, windy weather; morning; warmth; moisture; when touched; bright light.
Better: in the dark; coffee.

Primary Indicated Conditions

allergies   headaches
common cold   measles
conjunctivitis

EUPHRASIA

FERRUM PHOSPHORICA/Ferrum phos
(Common name: Phosphate of iron)

Overview

Ferrum phosphorica (Ferrum phos) was introduced into homeopathic practice by Dr. W. H. Schussler, a German physician who developed the cell salt theory of applying homeopathic medicines. (See *Magnesia phosphorica* for more details about the Schussler cell salts.) Due to the ability of ferrum (iron) to attract oxygen, the ferrum part of *Ferrum phos* helps to clear up local congestive conditions. The phosphorus part of this medicine acts upon tendencies of the body to bleed internally or externally.

Ferrum phos, like *Aconitum,* is considered a homeopathic vitamin C because it is so effective in treating the first stages of inflammatory conditions, especially colds, flus, sore throats, coughs, and ear infections. And because a homeopathic dose of a substance helps the body absorb the substance more efficiently, *Ferrum phos* is commonly used in iron deficiency anemic conditions.

General Characteristics

Like *Aconitum* and *Belladonna, Ferrum phos* is good for the initial stages of inflammatory conditions (before pus formation has begun). However, *Ferrum phos* does not have the same intensity of symptoms as these medicines. Children who need this medicine will not have the anxious restlessness as those who need *Aconitum,* nor will they be as inflamed as those who need *Belladonna. Ferrum phos* is generally indicated when a child is sick but does not have many individualizing symptoms. Except for some general weakness, the sick child will probably be in good spirits; he will talk and laugh as though he were completely healthy. In fact, some homeopaths prefer not to use this remedy in some cases, simply allowing the child's body to heal itself. If, however, the parents want to speed up the natural healing process, they can give this remedy.

The child who needs *Ferrum phos* usually has a facial pallor with a tendency to flush easily from excitement. There may also be a pallor of the mucous membranes.

The child is sluggish, mentally and physically. He is generally weak and is easily fatigued. He wants to be left alone and hates being around people who upset him. He may have a general feeling of malaise and indifference.

A child who needs *Ferrum phos* will tend to have ailments that begin after exposure to cold or after a loss of bodily fluids (sweat from overexertion, blood from an injury or from heavy menstrual bleeding).

As is relatively common during the initial stages of illness, the child has a poor appetite. He has a specific aversion to meat and milk and a desire for sour foods and stimulants. He may have a sour taste in his mouth when burping, and later may vomit undigested food. He may get a distended stomach after eating. He is chilly and is worse in the open air.

Keynote Symptoms

- For the initial stages of inflammation
- Black and blue marks after injury
- Flushing of the face
- General weakness

Modalities

Worse: early morning and at night; being touched, jarred or moved; standing; open air; after eating; cold drinks; right side of the body; cold (though some individual symptoms, such as headaches and toothaches, may be relieved by cold applications).
Better: gentle, slow motion.

FERRUM PHOSPHORICA/Ferrum phos

Primary Indicated Conditions

bedwetting	fever
common cold	headaches
cough	influenza
earache	sore throat

GELSEMIUM
(Common name: Yellow jasmine)

Overview

Yellow jasmine belongs to the *Loganaceae* plant family, the same family as the plants that make up *Nux vomica, Ignatia,* and *Spigelia.* It is a highly poisonous plant which contains two powerful chemicals, gelsemicine and gelseminine, which cause increasingly serious symptoms as the dose is increased. A toxic dose has a depressant action on motor neurons, causing great muscular weakness which tends to progress to paralysis. It also causes slowed respiration leading to general fatigue.

Its medicinal value was said to have been accidentally discovered by a Mississippi farmer who gathered and ate it, thinking it was something else. It almost killed him. Homeopathic physician and botanist Dr. Edwin Hale heard about this poisoning and did further testing of *Gelsemium* and discovered its important therapeutic effects.

General Characteristics

General physical and mental fatigue leads to a drowsy-looking child; symptoms may include half-open and glassy eyes, a partially flushed face, quivering eyelids, a relaxed and dropped jaw, and loss of power in the limbs. Her whole body, especially her extremities, may feel very heavy. The lips tend to be dry, even cracked.

GELSEMIUM

The child's mind, like the body, is limp. She feels listless, lazy, apathetic, and wants to be left alone. She makes no effort to do anything, especially anything new. She wants to stay in bed as much as possible, though she may actually be too tired to fall asleep and stay asleep.

In addition to general weakness, individual parts of her body may tremble or quiver: the hands tremble when she lifts something; the feet tremble when the child walks; the tongue quivers when she sticks it out. Even her voice may tremble.

She may also tremble from the chills, especially up and down her back. Her face and head may be hot but her extremities are cold. Her face is somewhat flushed, the lips are dusky, and her eyes reddened.

The child may have diarrhea or a headache from anticipation. This kind of anxiety is common in children before an examination, competitive game, a speech, or a performance. *Gelsemium* will often reduce this anxiety. It is also helpful for the child who is anticipating doing something that requires great courage. In addition, *Gelsemium* is also good for children who get sick after hearing bad news or after a sudden fright.

One of the child's characteristic symptoms, especially during the flu, is a lack of thirst, a quite unusual symptom considering that most people during fevers have an increased thirst. Despite the little thirst, the child may urinate profusely and will feel better afterward.

Gelsemium symptoms are known to begin quite slowly, distinct from *Aconitum* and *Belladonna*, which are medicines for colds and flus that have a very rapid onset of symptoms.

Keynote Symptoms

- Physical and mental weakness and exhaustion
- Heaviness of individual parts, especially eyelids and extremities

GELSEMIUM

- Listlessness, drowsiness, and apathy
- Trembling and quivering of individual parts
- Absence of thirst

Modalities

Worse: exposure to the sun; humid or damp weather; fog; 10:00 A.M.; emotion or excitement; bad news.
Better: warmth; after profuse urination; stimulants; open air.

Primary Indicated Conditions

anxiety	influenza
common cold	measles
headaches	

HEPAR SULPHURICUM/Hepar sulphur
(Common name: Hahnemann's Calcium Sulphide)

Overview

This medicine was initially conceived by homeopathy's founder Samuel Hahnemann. He mixed finely powdered oyster shells with elemental sulphur and burned the mixture for ten minutes at white heat. Hahnemann, who in addition to being a physician was a chemist and an avid experimenter, frequently tested various mixtures of substances. He developed *Hepar sulphur* from an oyster shell, which is the source of a major homeopathic medicine *Calcarea carbonica* (calcium carbonate), and *Sulphur,* another extremely common homeopathic remedy.

Typically, when two medicinal substances are mixed together, the mixture creates symptoms which are characteristic of both substances, though the majority of symptoms represents a new pattern unique to the newly created substance.

Hepar sulphur affects the nervous system, treating extremes of hypersensitivity and excitability, physically and psychologically. It also affects the skin and lymph system and is especially effective in treating skin infections in which there is much pus.

General Characteristics

Hepar sulphur is commonly given to children suffering from colds, coughs, sore throats, or ear infections, when the primary symptoms are aggravation from cold, sensitivity to touch, and irritable dispositions. If there are no other distinct symptoms to suggest another medicine, give *Hepar sulphur.*

A child who needs *Hepar sulphur* is hypersensitive, both physically and psychologically. He is extremely sensitive to touch, noise, pain, people, surroundings, even the wind. Simply combing his hair may hurt his head.

He is very irritable: touchy, quarrelsome, angry over trifles, difficult to please, impatient, and frequently hurried. He is also very sensitive to hearing bad news or to seeing someone in pain.

The *Hepar sulphur* condition usually includes profuse discharges of offensive and often sour-smelling pus, mucus, and sweat. Every little cut becomes infected and hypersensitive to touch and cold. The common cold and cough produce much mucus that rattles in the chest. The sweat is profuse, even on slight exertion.

The child is very chilly and is extremely sensitive to cold. He has a difficult time staying warm, and will go to great extents to keep his head warm. The child wants to stay at home during illness because of the comfort. The symptoms may begin after exposure to cold or will be worsened if even one part of the body gets chilled. He is also sensitive to dry weather and may feel some relief in wet or humid weather.

Typically, the child has pains as though a stick, fishbone, or plug were stuck in his throat, ear, or head. The boil or

HEPAR SULPHURICUM/Hepar sulphur

infected cut will be extremely sensitive to touch and cold. The skin will look unhealthy, sometimes yellowed, and the child will tend to have swollen lymph glands.

The sick child who will benefit from *Hepar sulphur* may have nausea, but will crave sour foods, specifically vinegar and pickles. He may also crave spicy foods and be averse to fatty foods. He usually is very thirsty.

Prescribing note: Using high potencies (200x and higher) of *Hepar sulphur* tends to prevent the formation of pus, while using lower potencies (12x and under) once pus has formed tends to speed up the process of discharge.

Keynote Symptoms

- Hypersensitive and excitable, physically and psychologically
- Very irritable, quarrelsome, and impatient
- Easy pus formation
- Splinterlike pains
- Offensive discharges and perspiration

Modalities

Worse: cold air; light touch; lying on the painful side; wind; morning; evening; night; winter; dry weather; uncovering the body.
Better: warmth; wet weather; after eating; wrapping up the head.

Primary Indicated Conditions

boils	croup
common cold	earache
cough	impetigo

HEPAR SULPHURICUM/Hepar sulphur

laryngitis   splinters
sinusitis   toothache
sore throat

HYPERICUM
(Common name: St. John's Wort)

Overview

King George VI of England (1895–1952) was so enamored of homeopathy and of the value of *Hypericum* in treating injuries that he named one of his prize racehorses Hypericum. The French call this herb *All-Holy* and the Irish call it *Mary's Glory*. The name *Hypericum* is derived from the Greek and means "over an apparition," in reference to the belief that this herb was so obnoxious to evil spirits that simply a whiff of it would cause them to leave.

Modern research has discovered many remarkable features of this herb: it has antiviral effects, antiseptic action, and it even has monoamine oxidase (MAO) inhibiting activity, known to be effective in treating depression. Although discussion of the treatment of AIDS is outside the scope of this book, research at New York University and the Weizmann Institute has shown that the tincture of St. John's Wort displays dramatic activity against the family of viruses that includes HIV.

The tincture of St. John's Wort is reddish in color, primarily due to a red pigment called hypericin in the plant. The *Doctrine of Signatures*, the medieval belief that the physical appearance of a plant reveals its healing virtues, suggests that red plants are good for wounds. Dr. Charles Millspaugh, the esteemed nineteenth-century botantist, noted that St. John's Wort was an invaluable treatment for wounds during the Civil

HYPERICUM

War. Modern research has verified folk wisdom, demonstrating that hypericin and other antibiotic chemicals in St. John's Wort help prevent wound infection.

In addition to these valuable external applications of St. John's Wort, internal homeopathic doses of it help speed the healing of wounds and are particularly effective in healing injuries to nerves.

General Characteristics

Called the *Arnica* of the nerves, *Hypericum* is a medicine *par excellence* for injuries to the nerves or to parts of the body rich with nerves. You can tell when there has been nerve injury when there are shooting pains or numbness.

Hypericum is great for treating crushed toes or fingers, concussions to the spine, especially the coccyx, and blows to the head. It is also effective for ailments after an injury to the nerves, such as a headache after a blow to the head, fall on the spine, or injury to the tongue. Phantom limb pains and convulsions after a head injury call for the use of *Hypericum*.

Virginia dentist and homeopath Dr. Richard Fischer uses *Hypericum* when children injure their front teeth, and states, "There are so many nerves in those front teeth that I have found that *Hypericum* works even better than *Arnica*."

Hypericum is also effective after an injury when a child has an impairment of memory or a tendency to make mistakes in writing.

Because many types of surgery traumatize nerves, *Hypericum* 6 or 30 should be given at least once before surgery and as needed afterward.

In addition to being effective for nerve injuries, *Hypericum* is helpful in treating simple punctures from nails, splinters, pins, and animal bites. *Hypericum* can be used internally and externally for these puncture wounds.

Hypericum is effective in external application for deep

HYPERICUM

wounds because it has the ability to help close them. Whereas *Calendula* is effective for superficial cuts, *Hypericum* is used for deeper and wider wounds as well as for gunshot wounds. If *Calendula* is used externally, you can give *Hypericum* internally at the same time.

Prescribing note: When using *Hypericum* tincture, make certain to dilute it with water. Because this tincture is 65 percent alcohol, you should dilute it approximately ten parts water to one part *Hypericum* tincture, or the child will be irritated by stinging.

Keynote Symptoms

- Injury to nerves or to parts of the body rich with nerves
- Shooting pains or headache after an injury
- Pre- and post-surgery when nerves are affected
- Bleeding hemorrhoids

Modalities

Worse: cold or damp weather; foggy weather; before a storm; touch or movement.
Better: keeping still; bending the head backward.

Primary Indicated Conditions

backache	headaches
birth trauma	head injuries
bites and stings	smashed fingers or toes
bruises	surgery
cuts	toothache

HYPERICUM

IGNATIA
(Common name: St. Ignatius Bean)

Overview

This herb was originally called St. Ignatius Bean by the Jesuits in China who, upon finding it to be a powerful medicine, named it after one of their saints. However, because it is also very poisonous, the Chinese, Jesuits, and ultimately homeopaths learned to use very small doses of it.

St. Ignatius Bean, like the plant from which *Nux vomica* is derived, contains strychnine. Due to this poison's toxic effects on the human nervous system, the medicine in homeopathic form is effective in treating various neurological complaints. Because of the deep connection between the human psyche and the nervous system, *Ignatia* is a very important medicine for ailments experienced after psychological stress.

General Characteristics

Ignatia is one of the most common medicines for ailments that begin after an emotional crisis. Children who can benefit from *Ignatia* get various physical symptoms after feeling grief, anxiety, or depression, and especially after someone close to them dies or even leaves them. It is typically used for sensitive, nervous, excitable children, more often girls than boys (boys are more commonly given *Nux vomica*, if and when the symptoms fit).

Initially, a child who needs *Ignatia* does not express her emotions, and she does not stick up for herself when she has been hurt. She holds in her anger, grief, or fear, then withdraws and pretends that everything is OK. She may accidentally expose her internal anxiety with trembling. She sighs often. Ultimately, she explodes into rage or hysteria.

This type of child is easily upset by trifles and easily of-

IGNATIA

fended. She is not, however, the type of child who gets and stays angry, nor is violent behavior a predominant characteristic. She generally feels misunderstood, and she rejects and is irritated by any sympathy.

Ignatia is a common medicine for a child who has been abused, either physically or emotionally. It is also a common remedy for adolescent and teenage girls who suffer from anorexia and bulimia.

Ignatia is also indicated for high-strung and sensitive children after they have been reprimanded. It is good for homesickness as well.

The moods of the child who needs *Ignatia* are changeable and contradictory: laughter and tears alternate or mingle; she may be very angry and then suddenly become remorseful and repentant; she may be rude and rebellious, then become docile. Her circulation is unstable, as shown by frequent changes in the color of the face (pallor alternating with easy flushing).

Writing about this kind of person, homeopathic psychiatrist Edward C. Whitmont said that the "overwrought state is the expression of [the patient's] desperate attempt to break free from the net in which he feels himself entangled." The person is entangled in contradictory physical symptoms: a hypersensitivity to pain that is worse by a light touch but is relieved by firm pressure; hunger that is not relieved by eating; sore throat pain that is relieved by swallowing; headache that is better from stooping.

The child may even have a paradoxical appetite: she will be repelled by an ordinary diet, warm food, and meat, but crave exotic foods and indigestible things. Older children may be irritated by coffee, but they may also be calmed by it. They also sometimes crave cold foods or drinks, bread, or sour things. They are often sensitive to tobacco smoke, which seems to suffocate them.

Like her emotions, which seem to get stuck in her throat

IGNATIA

and are left unexpressed, she tends to have a lump in her throat. Also, she sometimes has a sense of a lump or heaviness in her stomach after eating.

The child's overall nervousness may show itself in trembling, twitching, jerking, and a tendency to faint. She becomes so sensitive to every distraction and is so tangled in her various emotions that she often has difficulty sleeping.

Keynote Symptoms

- Ailments after grief, anxiety, or depression
- Ailments after embarrassment or scolding
- Emotional instability
- Much sighing or yawning
- Contradictory symptoms
- Sense of a lump in the throat or stomach

Modalities

Worse: emotional upset; unexpressed grief; suppressed depression; repressed anxiety; after hearing bad news; after disappointed love; cold; eating sweets; coffee; alcohol; tobacco smoke; strong odors; consolation; touch; before and during menstruation.

Better: warmth; while eating; by change of position; by pressure on the painful part; by activity which distracts the child.

Primary Indicated Conditions

anger	indigestion
anxiety	insomnia
grief	sore throat
headaches	

IGNATIA

IPECACUAHNA/Ipecac
(Common name: Ipecac root)

Overview

Ipecacuahna (Ipecac) derives its name from a Portuguese word for "road-side, sick-making plant." Wouldn't it be convenient if all herbs had such descriptive names in our own language? All parts of this plant are bitter, acrid, and nauseating to the taste. Even its odor is irritating enough that it can provoke a sneeze, and it occasionally elicits an asthmatic attack in sensitive people.

A toxic dose of ipecac has specific effects on the mucous lining of the digestive and respiratory tracts, creating increased secretion, spasms, and stimulating the vomiting center in the brain. It can also cause redness and blistering of the skin.

Ipecac in conventional medical doses is a well-known substance which physicians recommend having in home first-aid kits. Because it causes vomiting, it can be valuable, even life-saving, if a person accidentally swallows something poisonous. Because ipecac causes nausea and vomiting, homeopathically it is an important remedy for their cure. And because it causes redness of the skin, children with fevers will benefit from homeopathic doses of *Ipecac* when they have flushed faces. The tongue will be obviously more red than normal, and if there is bleeding, the blood will be bright rather than dark red.

General Characteristics

When the first symptom of illness is nausea which is not relieved by vomiting, or when nausea is the primary and persistent primary complaint, think of *Ipecac*.

Ipecac is indicated for nausea, whether there is vomiting or not. If there is vomiting, the child may either regurgitate food or simply experience empty retching. Commonly, he develops his symptoms after eating pork, veal, or rich foods such as pastries, ice cream, or sweets.

Despite the nausea, he will usually have a clean, uncoated tongue, and he may be thirstless. He will generally have an aversion and disgust for food, not only to smelling it but even to the thought of it. He may have cold perspiration, especially on his face.

Infants or children who need *Ipecac* tend to have profuse salivation and are constantly obliged to swallow their saliva. Drooling is a common symptom of infants who need *Ipecac*. They may also have much mucus secretion in their throats and bronchial tubes, causing them to cough. For some reason these children have a desire to put their fingers in their mouths.

The child's ill state brings out ill humor, impatience, and restlessness, though not to the same degree as the child who needs *Arsenicum*. Nothing pleases him, and he will yell and scream until he gets what he wants. Unfortunately, he doesn't always know what he wants, so he may yell and scream simply because he is irritable. Sometimes, his ailment begins after he has been vexed, embarrassed, or suppressed his anger. A child often experiences *Ipecac* states after being punished.

He is irritated by noise, especially music. He has restless sleep with vivid dreams. He is generally very chilly and weak.

Typically during indigestion, his face is pale, with a look typical of many children with nausea (sunken eyes, slightly open mouth).

Ipecac is also a key remedy for children who have frequent nosebleeds, especially when the blood is bright red.

Prescribing note: Arsenicum is sometimes a good medicine to give as a follow-up after *Ipecac* when another remedy is needed to complete a cure. A second medicine is needed when the child's symptoms change, still causing significant discomfort, and now more closely fitting another medicine.

IPECACUAHNA/Ipecac

Keynote Symptoms

- Persistent nausea and vomiting
- Profuse secretion and mucus
- Clean tongue
- Thirstless
- Hemorrhage

Modalities

Worse: food (especially veal and pork); motion; hot or humid weather; cold.
Better: rest with eyes closed.

Primary Indicated Conditions

asthma	diarrhea
bleeding	headaches
cough	indigestion

KALI BICHROMICUM/Kali Bic
(Common names: Potassium Bichromate, Bichromate of Potash)

Overview

Literally any substance can be made into a homeopathic medicine as long as you know what it causes in overdose. Because of this, homeopaths not only use substances from the plant, mineral, and animal kingdom but also various chemicals. The difference between homeopathic medicines and the chemicals used in conventional medicine is that homeopaths utilize considerably smaller and safer doses of the substance, and they prescribe them more individually—according to the person's total pattern of symptoms.

Potassium bichromate is obtained from chromium iron ore and is commonly used in fabric dyes, wood stains, photography, and electric batteries. It is both a corrosive irritant—a poison—and an oxidizing substance. When swallowed, it causes irritation, inflammation, and secretion of thick, stringy, mucousy discharges.

General Characteristics

Kali bic is most effective for a child with thick, stringy, tenacious mucus, either from the nose, eyes, throat, chest, or vagina. This tough and lumpy mucus sticks to the orifice and tends to be difficult to eliminate. If an acutely ill child has this type of discharge, *Kali bic* is often the indicated remedy.

The discharge is most commonly yellowish, though it may also be greenish. The child's skin tends to have a yellowish tint, and her vomit is predominantly yellow as well.

She usually feels listless, not wanting to make any physical or mental effort. She is averse to meeting new people and may not like people at all. Her digestion of food is similarly slow and listless. Although her nausea may be slightly relieved by eating, she usually feels worse overall afterward. She may get diarrhea shortly after eating, and the food feels as though it is lying like a load in her stomach. She may crave acid drinks, avoid meat, and be aggravated by coffee (or by a breast-feeding mother who drinks it).

These children are also known for having symptoms that migrate and alternate. The symptoms may move around the body, often from a specific small spot, one which your thumb could easily cover, to another spot. The symptoms may alternate too. For instance, a child's headache may disappear and be replaced with a nasal discharge or diarrhea.

The child tends to be chilly and prefers to wear a lot of

KALI BICHROMICUM/Kali Bic

clothing. She will be aggravated by cold weather and from being uncovered, but she will also tend to become ill after a change from cold to warm weather. Although her symptoms may be aggravated in the morning and night, her worst symptoms are sometimes at 2:00 A.M.

Kali bic is most typically indicated for light-haired, fat or chubby children and for stout teenagers, though it can be helpful for thin children when key symptoms match.

Keynote Symptoms

- Stringy, ropy, tenacious discharges, usually yellowish or greenish
- Pain at the root of the nose
- Alternating and migrating pains

Modalities

Worse: cold air, cold winds; open air; wet weather; being uncovered; touch; stooping; 2:00 A.M.; after waking from sleep; spring and autumn.
Better: warmth; motion; firm pressure; summer.

Primary Indicated Conditions

allergies	headaches
common cold	laryngitis
cough	measles
croup	sinusitis

LEDUM PALUSTRE/Ledum
(*Common names: Wild Rosemary, Marsh Tea*)

Overview

Wild rosemary (not the same species as the spice rosemary) has been used for several centuries. The Swedes used it to wash oxen and kill lice, and its branches were placed in grain to ward off mice. The Swedes also added it to their beer to increase its intoxicating effects.

Its leaves are narrow and lance-shaped. The leaves at the lower part of the plant are covered with soft downy hairs which enable the plant to conserve heat. This may explain its name, which is derived from the Greek word *ledos,* meaning "a woolen garment."

Wild rosemary is a member of the *Ericaceae* family, a family of plants known since ancient times. It grows in cold northern regions, usually in wet, marshy areas. Its flourishing in a cold environment is mirrored homeopathically, as people who need *Ledum* feel relief from cold or cold applications. Whether it is from an animal bite, insect sting, injury, or inflammation, *Ledum* is an important medicine to consider when relief of pain is obtained with cold applications.

The flowers have a strong odor because of an antiseptic, camphorlike oil, ledol. Bees are attracted to the flowers, but they do not usually land on them due to the flower's poisonous nature. (It is interesting that *Ledum* is also used in homeopathy for beestings.)

The plant's medicinal action heals muscles and connective tissues after injury or inflammation and also cleanses the blood after an animal bite or insect sting.

General Characteristics

Ledum is the primary remedy for puncture wounds and for bites and stings. Dr. Adolph Teste, a contemporary of homeopathy's founder Samuel Hahnemann, noted that *Ledum,* like *Arnica,* helps to heal bruises because of its action on capillaries. *Ledum,* however, is particularly effective in treating the smaller capillaries, thus making it valuable for treating bruises to the hands and feet.

Ledum is the best medicine for healing black eyes, and it helps a variety of bruises, especially when *Arnica* has

LEDUM PALUSTRE/Ledum

provided some benefit but hasn't sufficiently cured the condition. It is indicated for long-lasting bruises. Most typically, the bruises are relieved by cold, cold applications, and cold bathing.

Ledum is the primary medicine for treating bites and stings from mosquitoes, bees, spiders, and rats. It helps to reduce itching and inflammation.

A child who needs *Ledum* may be cold, though she is aggravated by heat and relieved by cold.

Ledum also effectively treats skin rashes caused by poison ivy, oak, or sumach, especially when the symptoms are relieved by cold applications. *Ledum* can also be used as a way to prevent a skin rash after being exposed to the plant. Jacquelyn Wilson, M.D., former president of the American Institute of Homeopathy, tells the story of a four-year-old girl who picked a bouquet of poison oak leaves, nice and red, and gave the bouquet to her mother. Even though mother and daughter were normally hypersensitive to poison oak, neither got any rash whatsoever, thanks to an immediate dose of *Ledum* 30.

Ledum is also effective in treating sprains of various sorts, though it is most effective in curing children who sprain their ankles easily.

Keynote Symptoms

- Puncture wounds
- Black eyes and bruises
- Bites and stings
- Sprained ankle
- Pain relieved by cold applications

Modalities

Worse: heat; heat of bed; being dressed too warmly; motion; at night.

LEDUM PALUSTRE/Ledum

Better: cold; cold applications; cold bathing; rest.

Primary Indicated Conditions

bites and stings	poison ivy, oak, or sumach
bruises	puncture wounds
eye injuries	sprains and strains

MAGNESIA PHOSPHORICA/Mag Phos
(Common name: Phosphate of magnesium)

Overview

Phosphate of magnesium is an inorganic mineral in the blood, muscles, brain, spinal marrow, nerves and teeth. It is one of the twelve tissue salts (also called *cell salts*) described by Dr. W. H. Schussler, a German homeopathic physician who developed a system of prescribing these remedies for a wide variety of human ills. Dr. Schussler suggested that disease resulted from an imbalance in the tissue salts and that homeopathic potentized doses of these substances could correct the imbalances. Today, we know that the human body is dependent upon the balance and interaction of thousands of biochemical processes, not just twelve. Despite Schussler's simplistic views, homeopaths have found that these medicines are invaluable remedies for various conditions.

Mag phos is known to affect nervous and muscular tissues and helps to cure neuralgic pains and muscle spasms.

General Characteristics

Mag phos and *Colocynthis* are two of the primary remedies for colic, cramps, or spasms that are relieved by heat, bending double, and pressure. It is predictable that these two medicines would have some common symptoms, considering that *Colocynthis* contains some *Mag phos.*

Quite distinct from the angry and irritable types of children who need *Colocynthis,* children who will benefit from *Mag phos* are not given to fits of rage. The child tends to be averse to mental effort and instead prefers to be quiet, remain warm, covered, and bent double.

The child feels relief from warmth, warm drinks, warm applications, and the warmth of a bed, and feels worse when exposed to the cold. *Mag phos* is a primary remedy for teenage girls who get abdominal or premenstrual uterine cramps.

Mag phos is useful for cramps, stiffness, or numbness after prolonged writing, musical instrument playing, or manual labor. The pains may be induced by overexertion or from the prolonged use of certain muscles.

Children who need *Mag phos* may have cramping, shooting, excruciating pains. Rarely will they get burning pains. Sometimes their pains begin after exposure to cold or cold damp weather. The pains come and go suddenly, and they may be so severe that they cause retching.

When the child has abdominal cramps, she may also have bloating which is not relieved by the passing of gas.

Mag phos is indicated for teething infants when warm or hot drinks or applications provide relief.

Keynote Symptoms

- Cramps relieved by heat or warm applications; bending double; firm pressure

- Cramps aggravated by cold or cold applications

Modalities

Worse: cold; cold wind; cold water; cold draught; touch; movement; night.

MAGNESIA PHOSPHORICA/Mag Phos

Better: warmth; warm applications; pressure or rubbing; bending double; rest.

Primary Indicated Conditions

backache   teething
colic

MERCURIUS
(Common name: Mercury)

Overview

Despite the fact that mercury has long been known to be highly poisonous, it was a very popular medicine in the fifteenth century due to its reputation for treating syphilis. Mercury was known as a purgative and a cathartic, which means that it stimulated bowel function and vomiting and therefore helped rid the body of undesirable substances. Mercury also leads to the production of much salivation, hence the saying associated with what was once thought to be a cure of syphilis: "Salivation is salvation."

Mercury, however, creates its own set of serious problems, and can make people die more rapidly from mercury poisoning than from syphilis. Ironically (but predictably), mercury in overdose causes ulceration, a chancrelike symptom. Homeopaths assume that the reason that mercury helps to temporarily reduce the symptoms of syphilis is that it also causes syphilitic symptoms.

Mercury is quite an extraordinary substance. It is a liquid at room temperature and evaporates easily. It is very sensitive to temperature, hence its great value in thermometers. It is fitting that the sick children who will benefit from *Mercurius* are those who are similarly sensitive to extremes of temperature. Their symptoms are aggravated by both heat and cold.

MERCURIUS

In Roman mythology, Mercury was the messenger of the Gods. Perhaps, then, it is no coincidence that homeopathic *Mercurius* can help people communicate better: it is one of the primary remedies for those who stammer or speak too hastily.

General Characteristics

Mercurius is effective in treating advanced stages of acute conditions—including diarrhea and sore throat—with strong pain and profuse, offensive, burning, and bloody discharges. It is also the most commonly given remedy for children with chronic ear infections.

Hypersensitivity to both hot and cold indicates a need for *Mercurius.* The child tends to be chilly but will feel worse in a warm room and from the warmth of the bed. He may have hot and cold sensations that will alternate or be aggravated after a change in the weather. He may be easily chilled, from even just touching something cold. The open air or a cold wind will chill him to the bone, and yet later he may experience flashes of heat.

Perhaps the most common symptom to call for this remedy is profuse salivation. The child wets his pillow or slobbers or gulps his own saliva. He has a dry throat despite his increased salivation. He will also have an intense thirst despite having a moist mouth. This thirst is primarily for cold drinks, especially milk or soda pop. He usually has an insatiable hunger, though he could also be averse to all foods. If he is hungry, he usually won't want meat, and when ill, he won't want sweets. He may crave butter, or he may be disgusted at the thought of it.

Not only does this child salivate profusely, he perspires profusely, usually an offensive, oily sweat. Although most children feel better after perspiring, a child who needs *Mercurius* doesn't. In fact, he may feel exhausted during and after sweating. He also has smelly discharges and bad breath.

The child is restless and can't stay still, though he becomes

MERCURIUS

easily exhausted as well. He experiences a weakness of the mind, difficulty concentrating, irritability, and mental depression. This weakness is also seen in his body; he trembles from the least exertion, especially of his hands, or simply when he sticks out his tongue.

Typically, a child who needs *Mercurius* gets colds that settle in his throat. Due to the advanced stage of his inflammatory condition, he tends to have swollen lymph glands. He may also have a pale, flabby tongue that may have the imprint of his teeth.

The symptoms tend to be worse at night and are aggravated when the child lies on the right side.

Keynote Symptoms

- Symptoms made worse by extremes of temperature

- Symptoms worse at night and in wet weather

- Profuse, offensive, and burning discharges

- Excession salivation

- Profuse and constant perspiration

Modalities

Worse: extremes of temperature; change in the weather; open air; evening and night; touch and pressure; after eating; during and after perspiration; after exertion.
Better: during the day; from rest; at high altitudes.

Primary Indicated Conditions

canker sores	hepatitis
cold sores	mumps
conjunctivitis	sore throat
diarrhea	thrush
earache	toothache
food poisoning	

MERCURIUS

NUX VOMICA
(Common name: Poison nut)

Overview

The poison nut tree is an evergreen of the *Loganiaceae* family, similar to the family to which St. Ignatius Bean (*Ignatia*) belongs. Homeopaths use the seeds from this tree which, like St. Ignatius Bean, contain strychnine, a poisonous alkaloid that has powerful effects upon the nervous system. It is poisonous to virtually every animal and bird except cats and snails. It causes initial excessive excitement of the nervous system and all the senses, and creates muscle spasms that later lead to exhaustion and paralysis.

The poison nut tree has a crooked trunk and irregular, awkward-looking branches. Its flowers bloom in the cold season and have a disagreeable odor—characteristics contrary to most flowers which bloom in the warm season and have a pleasant odor.

These contrary features are characteristic of children who need *Nux vomica* as well. They are chilly, both physically and psychologically. They are disagreeable, irritable, and quarrelsome.

Homeopaths find that *Nux vomica* more often fits the symptoms of boys than girls, while *Ignatia* more often fits the symptoms of girls than boys, though either of these medicines can be given to both sexes. *Nux vomica,* for instance, should be used when the girl is a very competitive type and suffers from the typical *Nux* symptoms described here.

General Characteristics

Nux vomica is a classic medicine for the modern day. It is the most common remedy for ailments that arise from overindulgence in rich foods, alcohol, or drugs (or from the mother's use or abuse of these during pregnancy or breast-feeding). It is indicated for the child who suffers from complaints after a bout of anger, after prolonged mental stress at home or school, or after disappointment at not reaching a personal goal.

Children who need *Nux vomica* are hyperactive and over-excitable. Dr. Margery Blackie, the late physician to Queen Elizabeth II, described a child who benefits from *Nux vomica* as "causing reactions," often throwing tantrums at home or in public and then wildly fending off anyone who tries to stop him. He thrives on rebellion. As the child enters adolescence, he becomes one of the first kids to smoke or drink.

But this rebelliousness also demonstrates the child's self-reliance. He tends to be a driven individual who works hard and fast and expects others to work as zealously as he does. He is a competitive child, both with his siblings and with his friends. He is full of zeal but full of worries too. He is often tense and overanxious. He is irritated by the slightest stress, quarrelsome, fault-finding, and impatient. His irritability and impatience is often expressed by his demand to be cured of his illness immediately.

He is fastidious and is especially fussy about order and accuracy. Even when he is ill, he will want his room in order, and will want to know the precise number of homeopathic pellets to take.

His revved-up nervous system makes him sensitive to touch, pain, noise, odors, music, food, and drugs. He is a light sleeper, and angry at whoever wakes him up. He gets particularly irritable if he doesn't get enough sleep.

The child also gets bloated and flatulent; it is usually worse about one hour after eating, especially after eating meat, milk, or cold food. The child may have other symptoms after these foods as well, including headaches and respiratory conditions. He desires fats and spicy foods. He tends to be constipated and has frequent, ineffectual urgings for a stool—as distinct from a constipated child who has no urgings at all.

NUX VOMICA

A headache along with nausea and a loathing of food may accompany the child's constipation. The head pain is worse in the morning and from any exertion. It begins while the child is in bed and is worse from stooping, light, noise, exposure to the sun, moving or opening the eyes, and from coughing. Some relief is experienced from warmth, quiet, and pressure on the head.

Concurrent with a headache, indigestion, or emotional upset, the child needing *Nux vomica* may also have a fluent nasal discharge during the day and congestion at night. These respiratory symptoms will tend to be worse indoors, especially in a warm room, and are better in the open air. They are made worse by exposure to the cold and by being uncovered. The child is especially sensitive to dry, cold weather and sometimes will feel better in moist or wet weather.

He is worse upon waking, worse at night, at midnight, and between 3:00 A.M. and 4:00 A.M.

He gets cramps in his extremities and various twitchings and jerkings in his muscles.

Keynote Symptoms

- Complaints after overindulgence in food, alcohol, or stimulants

- Complaints after prolonged mental or emotional stress

- Very irritable

- Frequent, ineffectual urgings for a stool

Modalities

Worse: by overindulgence in food (especially spicy or fatty foods); after drug use (recreational or therapeutic); after prolonged mental or emotional stress; cold or windy weather; in-

NUX VOMICA

sufficient sleep or from being aroused during sleep; noise; light; touch.

Better: rest; unbroken sleep; firm pressure; wet weather.

Primary Indicated Conditions

allergies	fever
anger	food poisoning
asthma	headaches
backache	hepatitis
colic	hives
common cold	indigestion
constipaton	insomnia
diarrhea	nervous restlessness

PHOSPHORUS
(Common name: Phosphorus)

Overview

Phosphorus is an essential element in both animal and plant life; it is necessary for a cell's energy production, storage, and release. It is also an essential nutrient in bones and teeth.

Phosphorus is widely available in foods, especially in sodas and food additives, and a deficiency of it in a child is very rare. The more common problem is excessive intake of this mineral, which can disrupt the delicately balanced chemistry of the body. For instance, too much phosphorus can cause the body to excrete excessive amounts of calcium. Due to the importance of phosphorus in so many physiological processes and due to its effect on other vital minerals in the body, it is a common and important homeopathic medicine.

Phosphorus is also known for giving off light without heat when exposed to air. Similar to phosphorescent light, a child who benefits from *Phosphorus* radiates an extroverted personality. Like a match with a phosphorus tip, he emits light but tends to burn out quickly and become exhausted.

A plant deficient in phosphorus develops a thin, long stem and weak roots. Similarly, a child who needs *Phosphorus* tends to be thin and tall, and not psychologically grounded. He tends to be off in his own world, has difficulty finishing projects, and is easily fatigued.

General Characteristics

Phosphorus is a common homeopathic medicine for a wide range of both acute and chronic conditions. It is most successfully prescribed based on the overall characteristics, rather than on just individual symptoms.

A child who needs *Phosphorus* is usually extroverted, even bubbly. He is full of life and mirth. He is fun to be with and is wonderfully entertaining. He truly loves being the center of attention. As much as he likes other people, he is also greatly influenced by them. He tends to be worried if they are worried, at ease if they are at ease, particularly in matters of health—his own and of those around him.

This type of child has a sympathetic nature; he wants company, attention, affection, and sympathy. He loves to be massaged, both because it feels good and because of the attention and affection that comes with it.

In the book *Psyche and Substance*, psychiatrist and homeopath Edward C. Whitmont describes the person who needs *Phosphorus* to be like a delicate blossom that "thrives in the sunshine of favorable circumstances but wilts in the darkness of coldness of adversity."

Besides being emotionally impressionable, the child is also strongly affected by his physical environment. He is sensitive to cold (he may become ill shortly after being chilled), changes of temperature (he sometimes seems to be a human thermometer), odors (he is hypersensitive to perfume and tobacco), strong light (his eyes may hurt), and noise (he is easily startled).

Typically, this type of child has acute senses. Not only is he able to see, hear, and feel more than other children, but he sometimes is intuitive and can even be clairvoyant.

The child is susceptible to various fears, including fear of the dark, of being alone, of ghosts, of his illness, of thunder, and of spiders. Underneath these fears is usually a foreboding sense that something bad is going to happen to him. Being the expressive type of child that he is, he cannot help but talk about his fears and does so in dramatic fashion. Although his fears are easily provoked, they are also easily calmed by sympathetic attention. Because of the degree of personal, individual attention used in homeopathy, this type of child loves the homeopathic interview.

The fears are often felt in the body and usually in the pit of the stomach. The child may get diarrhea and will tremble from the slightest cause. Because of his various fears, he does not like to sleep alone, especially when feeling ill. If he can't sleep with his parents, he will ask to have a light turned on. Because of his impressionability, it isn't a good idea to read a scary bedtime story to this kind of child, or to let him see a violent or scary televion show before bedtime.

The child is also easily distracted. He has a short attention span, will get tired of toys quickly, and has difficulty paying attention in school. The positive side of this is that his fears can be temporarily relieved by drawing something more positive to his attention.

The child may become restless and fidget constantly and also have a tendency to flush easily. Although the child is usually chilly, he tends to have burning pains, commonly in the head, throat, chest, or abdomen. Most of the symptoms are relieved by warmth, except for headaches, which are aggravated by it.

Despite this chilliness, the child has a strong craving for cold food and ice drinks. He enjoys chewing on ice and loves

PHOSPHORUS

ice cream. He also craves salt, spicy foods, sweets, chocolate, bubble gum, and cold milk, and dislikes eggs, bread, fish, meat, boiled milk, tea, and sometimes sweets (except ice cream).

A child who needs *Phosphorus* tends to be frequently ill and to get recurrent infections, especially colds and coughs. He is also susceptible to frequent nosebleeding. Despite having an overall high level of energy, he is easily fatigued. He usually has a big appetite shortly before going to bed. The child more often has complaints on his left side, and has difficulty sleeping on this side.

Keynote Symptoms

- Burning pains, better by warmth (except headaches)
- Craves cold food and ice drinks
- Craves sympathy and company
- Chilly
- Very impressionable; very sensitive to their environment

Modalities

Worse: cold (except headaches); left side of the body; lying on the left side; odors; light; touch; sudden change in weather; during sunset; in the dark; before and during a thunderstorm.
Better: warmth; eating; cold food or drinks; sympathy; massage.

Primary Indicated Conditions

anxiety	hepatitis
bleeding	indigestion
cough	laryngitis
croup	nosebleed
headaches	

PHOSPHORUS

PODOPHYLLUM
(Common names: Podophyllum, May Apple)

Overview

Podophyllum was used by American Indians to help eliminate worms. They also used it when someone had ingested something poisonous, because its herbal doses help to flush poison out of the body. It is an irritant and corrosive wherever it is applied.

These properties have brought it to the attention of contemporary physicians. Podophyllin, a conventional drug taken from the dried extract of podophyllum, is painted on warts to burn them off. Its caustic properties also make it helpful in chemical face peels.

Experiments by homeopaths have discovered that toxic doses of podophyllum have a strong affinity to the liver when taken internally. Its caustic properties cause profuse, offensive diarrhea as well.

General Characteristics

Podophyllum is one of the most common medicines for diarrhea, especially when the diarrhea is profuse and foul-smelling. The diarrhea is commonly worse in the early morning (4:00 A.M. to 10:00 A.M.) and on hot summer days. *Podophyllum* is also useful for treating diarrhea in an infant during teething.

The diarrhea tends to be gushing, and the child's abdomen gurgles. She may have diarrhea when she thinks that she is only going to pass gas. This problem usually occurs when the child is suffering from food poisoning. The child has profuse, watery stools that literally shoot out. After this painless diarrhea, the child feels exhausted.

She tends to have an empty, sinking feeling in the abdomen after a stool. She may feel a sense of flabbiness in the

PODOPHYLLUM

internal organs. In particular, her liver may feel swollen and sensitive to touch, but feels better when rubbed. She may also have heartburn, nausea, and vomiting with a headache. The diarrhea may alternate with constipation.

The child may have offensive breath and a white-coated tongue with a funny taste in her mouth. She wants sour foods, if she wants food at all. She craves citrus fruits even though they aggravate her condition. She usually is very thirsty for cold drinks.

Podophyllum is often chosen for infants with diarrhea. They usually have profuse, offensive green stools. Their diarrhea may be so runny that it runs through the diaper. These infants roll their heads back and forth and try to press their gums together. They are restless and don't sleep well.

Keynote Symptoms

- Profuse, offensive diarrhea
- Worse in the early morning
- Worse during hot summer days
- Worse during teething

Modalities

Worse: in the morning, between 2:00 A.M. and 4:00 A.M.; hot weather; during teething; citrus fruits; milk, after eating; before, during, and after passing stools.
Better: rubbing or stroking the liver; lying on the abdomen; in the evening.

Primary Indicated Conditions

diarrhea

PODOPHYLLUM

PULSATILLA
(Common name: Windflower)

Overview

The windflower plant has characteristics in nature that are similar to the type of child for whom the medicine *Pulsatilla* is prescribed. The windflower grows in clusters, never alone; likewise, this type of child hates to be alone and is hungry for company. The windflower grows in dry sandy soil; the child similarly needs very little water and seems to never be thirsty. The windflower has a small, delicate, and flexible stem that bends in the wind, and it gets its name because its pollen are easily carried by the wind; the child is similarly gentle, mild, and yielding. She is flexible and adapts to her environment and, like the wind, is changeable and moody.

No other homeopathic medicine is prescribed more often for acute conditions in infants and children than *Pulsatilla*. When you read its general characteristics, you will probably easily recognize this type of child; you may even recognize yourself, a sibling, or a friend from childhood.

General Characteristics

There are so many indications for *Pulsatilla*—which is more commonly given to women and children than to men—that it is considered the Queen of Homeopathic Medicines. (*Sulphur* is the King.)

This child is an emotional, sensitive one. She is easily hurt, discouraged, swayed, weepy, and easily affected by people and her environment. She can cry for almost any reason, but especially if she is criticized or punished or if she is simply ignored. She never sobs; her crying has a sweet and innocent quality that makes you want to hug her. She is moody and may be weepy one moment and laugh the next. Once the child gets the

PULSATILLA

attention and sympathy she needs, her pain disappears and is quickly forgotten. She may even feign illness to get attention, or regress to baby talk and infant behavior in order to get extra nurturing. She soaks up affection and cannot get enough of it.

Infants want, even need, to be held; she is content only when she is picked up. She also cries whenever her parents leave her or if she has to sleep in her own bed, instead of with her parents.

The child has fears of abandonment and can be very clingy and whiny. She often becomes jealous of her siblings and wants more attention from her parents. Distinct from other kinds of children, however, she will not develop a full-blown temper tantrum, though her continued whining shows that she has an obstinate side, an aspect of her personality that comes out in order to get the attention she wants. On the rare occasions that she gets angry, it doesn't last for very long.

The child eagerly seeks to please others, usually as a way to get attention and affection. She is also an impressionable child. If, for instance, she is told a ghost story just prior to bedtime, she will have difficulty falling asleep or staying asleep. Whether she has been recently frightened or not, she often prefers to sleep with the light on, and she ends up in her parents' bed sometime in the night.

She is prone to self-pity, asking herself, "Why does this always happen to me?" This self-pity is also expressed in the feeling that she is not worthy of being loved.

The child has great difficulty making decisions, both important and trivial ones. If somebody doesn't make a decision for her, she often makes decisions by default: one of her choices inevitably becomes impossible due to her delay in decision making.

The child's physical symptoms are like her moody and changeable nature. She has wandering pains, changing symptoms, and pains that alternate sides of the body.

PULSATILLA

She is chilly but does not like hot weather. She can, in fact, become almost limp in hot weather. She hates warm rooms and high humidity. She dislikes covers and kicks them off, though she then wakes up when she gets too cold. She craves open air and coolness, but can't stand to be chilled. She may become ill after being chilled, especially after working up a sweat during play.

Pulsatilla is the most commonly indicated homeopathic medicine for children who develop digestive symptoms after eating too much rich or fatty food. Typically, the child returns home from a party after eating too much birthday cake holding her stomach and seeking sympathy. Although she craves ice cream, pastries, peanut butter, sweets, and rich foods, these foods tend to cause indigestion and other problems. She is averse to warm foods, fruits, milk, butter, and meat, especially pork and sausage. She is usually not thirsty, even if she has a fever. You generally have to force her to drink because she has very little desire for fluids.

This type of child gets frequent colds and coughs. Most typically, she has a thick, yellow or greenish discharge. The nasal congestion is usually worse at night or in a warm room; the nose gets congested when she lies down to sleep, making her breathe through her mouth. Like the child's changing emotional nature, the nasal congestion also tends to change, alternating sides.

Prescribing note: Pulsatilla is commonly prescribed based on its general characteristics rather than simply the local symptoms of a specific condition.

Keynote Symptoms

- Emotional, sensitive, moody children who crave attenton and sympathy
- Symptoms are worse in a warm or stuffy room or in hot weather and are relieved in the open air

PULSATILLA

- Symptoms begin after eating rich or fatty foods
- Lack of thirst

Modalities

Worse: heat; humidity; warm rooms; being chilled; the evening or first part of the night; ice cream; pastries; rich foods; hot food and drinks; evening and night.
Better: being in the open air; gentle motion; cold food; cool applications; lying on the painful side.

Primary Indicated Conditions

asthma	German measles
bedwetting	grief
colic	headaches
common cold	hives
conjunctivitis	impetigo
cough	insomnia
cystitis	measles
diarrhea	mumps
earache	sinusitis
fever	styes

RHUS TOXICODENDRON/Rhus tox
(Common name: Poison ivy)

Overview

Poison ivy and oak are restless plants that spread over countrysides. They do not simply stay in one place but cover increasingly more and more territory, either trailing along the ground or climbing up trees or other plants. Children who need *Rhus tox* are similarly restless, always on the go, both during waking hours and while tossing and turning during sleep.

RHUS TOXICODENDRON/Rhus tox

Although this plant is best known for causing irritating skin rashes in most of us who touch it, other animals do not have a similar sensitivity. Horses, mules, and goats eat the plant, and birds feast on its berries.

A peculiarity of this plant is that the active agent that causes the skin irritation, toxicodendric acid, increases in potency at night, during damp or cloudy weather, and in June and July. Some of these unique characteristics are mimicked in those children who need homeopathic doses of this plant: their symptoms are noticeably worse at night and in cold, damp weather. (Although *Rhus tox* is made from poison ivy, its symptoms are basically identical to those of poison oak *Rhus diversiloba* or sumac.)

General Characteristics

Like the restless growth of the poison ivy and oak plants, infants and children who will benefit from *Rhus tox* are also restless, usually so restless that they can't keep still. They are always moving and searching for comfortable positions that afford them relief.

This type of child is known to experience the *rusty-gate syndrome:* they feel stiff and aching, a condition worsened on initial motion and better from continued motion. It is almost as if the continued motion enables the body to, in some way, oil its joints so that they are not so stiff. Eventually, however, the child must sit or rest, but the pains come back during this time, and the rusty-gate syndrome is again experienced upon initial motion. This cycle of irritation during rest, aggravation during first motion, relief from continued motion, fatigue from exertion, and irritation from rest plays out recurrently.

The child is also very chilly and is aggravated by cold or wet weather. He may even become ill after getting chilled or wet, especially if this happens when he is overheated during play or exertion. He will be made worse by being uncovered, and his symptoms are usually worse at night.

RHUS TOXICODENDRON/Rhus tox

The child's sleep is predictably restless since many of the symptoms are aggravated during rest and at night. The child has difficulty finding the right position in which to fall asleep. He tosses and turns during sleep and may wake up, either because of the pain or to go to the bathroom. He will go through his rusty-gate syndrome again when he gets up.

A child benefited by *Rhus tox* usually has dry and cracked lips, often with a herpes blister. He craves cold drinks, especially at night, even though the cold drinks sometimes make him chillier and aggravate his cough. He has a special desire for milk, but usually does not have an appetite.

Children who need *Rhus tox* may become stiff after using muscles that have not been used in a long time. They may also get sick after overexerting themselves.

Keynote Symptoms

- Aggravation of symptoms from rest and on initial motion
- Relief of symptoms from continued motion
- Aggravation of symptoms at night and from cold or wet weather
- Restless, with much tossing and turning

Modalities

Worse: from initial motion; rest; cold; cold and wet weather; night; during sleep; overexertion; touch; scratching; bathing.
Better: from continued motion; warm covering.

Primary Indicated Conditions

backache	cold sores
chickenpox	hives

RHUS TOXICODENDRON/Rhus tox

impetigo

influenza

insomnia

mumps

poison ivy or oak

sore throat

sprain or strain

RUTA
(Common name: Rue)

Overview

The herb rue is one of the oldest cultivated garden plants in England. In the early days of Rome, rue was thought to make a warrior invincible if he heated his sword-point and spread the juice of the plant on it. Since *Ruta* is a great homeopathic medicine for injuries, this ritual offers an intriguing mythic connection.

Along with garlic, rue was one of the most common plants used to protect against evil. Rue was one of the herbs people used to ward off the plague. It has also been believed to impart second-sight. Although there is no scientific proof of its ability to restore vision, there are numerous reports about it being of value for the eyes. Ancient Roman naturalist Pliny reported that painters of his day regularly ate rue to restore overstrained eyes. Homeopaths today use *Ruta* for people who strain their eyes from reading too much.

General Characteristics

Ruta is the primary remedy for injuries to the periosteum (bone covering) or for bruises that heal slowly and leave a hardened spot. Such injuries usually occur at the knee, shin, or elbow. When there is a knotty lump (a ganglion) after an injury, *Ruta* should be considered. These ganglions often occur at the wrist. *Carpal tunnel syndrome,* which often occurs at

RUTA

the wrist in which lumpy bands of tissue form in the connective tissue, is usually cured by *Ruta*. Carpal tunnel syndrome is an increasingly common condition in children as a result of repeated wrist motions, such as from frequent use of a video game or computer keyboard.

Ruta should also be used before and after surgery on joints like the knee, elbow, wrist, or teeth. (Although most people do not think of teeth as joints, anatomists consider them to be ball and socket joints.) *Ruta* is extremely effective in reducing pain and in speeding healing after dental surgery.

Dr. Richard Fischer, a dentist in Annandale, Virginia, has repeatedly observed the benefits of *Ruta* after a tooth has been extracted. Along with *Arnica*, *Ruta* sharply reduces the post-operative pain. Dr. Fischer also notes that it is great for kids after they get their braces tightened or after orthodontists put spacers between the teeth in preparation for placing the orthodontic bands of braces.

Ruta, along with *Rhus tox*, are the two most common remedies for sprains. *Ruta* has a special affinity for injuries to the knee and elbow and to the surrounding tissue. It is the most common remedy for recurrent tennis elbow and chronic knee injuries.

Overstraining of muscles from overexertion or from repetitious motion that leads to an inflammatory condition may require *Ruta*, especially when *Arnica* or *Rhus tox* is not effective. The injured part will feel hot to the touch.

Prescribing note: *Arnica* and *Ruta* can be given together or individually pre- and post-operatively. If you choose to give them individually, consider giving *Arnica* just prior to the surgery and immediately after; then, give *Ruta* starting one or two hours after the surgery, depending on the pain. The greater the pain, the earlier you should give it, and the greater the pain after the first couple of hours, the more frequently the child should take it.

RUTA

Keynote Symptoms

- Injury to the periosteum (the bone covering)
- Injury or surgery to the knee, elbow, or teeth
- Injury to the tendons and ligaments

Modalities

Worse: lying on the painful part.
Better: warmth.

Primary Indicated Conditions

bone injuries	surgery
bruises	toothache
sprains and strains	

SILICEA
(Common names: Silica, Silicon dioxide)

Overview

Silica is second to oxygen as the most abundant element on this planet. Also known as silicon dioxide, silica appears in nature in quartz, flint, sandstone, sand, and numerous other minerals. It is a primary ingredient in cement and glass. Silica is also the ingredient in a blade of grass or a stalk of grain that helps it stand erect.

Silica has a similarly cohesive effect on the human body. Physiologists say that silica apears to be an essential element in the human body. Although there are only relatively small amounts of it in the body, collagen, the substance that holds tissue together, is high in silica. Arteries, tendons, skin, connective tissue, hair, nails, and eyes also contain large amounts of silica.

SILICEA

Various forms of silica are used in modern technology in radio transmitters, computer chips, and body implants. Silica's inert and nonreactive nature are exhibited by its water repellence and its resistance to heat and oxidation, characteristics that make it invaluable in today's technological world. Children who benefit from *Silicea* are those who may, like a computer chip, store information, but do not have the self-confidence, the psychological collegen, to stand up for themselves to impart it. Their nonreactive nature is exhibited by their tendency to complacently vegetate as the world moves around them.

General Characteristics

These infants or children develop their symptoms slowly, and those who need this remedy will respond to the medicine in a similarly slow manner.

The child is also physically and emotionally slow. He is easily fatigued and becomes pale after simple exertion. He lacks drive and grit. He is also very shy and has a fear of doing new things because he fears failure. Although he lacks confidence in his abilities, he is actually quite bright and usually does things well if he can finish them. Like a blade of grass without silica, a child who needs this remedy does not stand up for himself and wilts unless he is given much encouragement.

The child is easily startled and easily irritated by little things. Sometimes these little things upset him more than big things. His obsession, in this respect, may show itself in a fear of pins. Although he may hunt for pins and count them, he is ultimately afraid of them.

The child can be very stubborn, though he won't be aggressive or argumentative. Instead, he will be pleasant, doing what he wants in his own way.

Like the child's shy personality, his stools are similarly bashful—partially expelled but then slipping back into the

SILICEA

rectum. The child can get so constipated that he has great difficulty in having a stool at all, even a soft stool. In extreme cases, he will hardly ever feel the urge to defecate.

The child is usually cold, sallow-looking, and sweaty. He typically has a large head, protruding belly, and a small body. He sweats profusely on the head and feet.

His lack of energy makes him extremely chilly. Part of the problem is that he has a poor appetite and poor assimilation of food. Strangely enough, he wants to eat indigestible objects such as dirt, sand, or hair. If he is hungry, he craves cold foods and drinks and is averse to warm foods. He will either crave milk or loathe it. He may get diarrhea or colic from his mother's milk. Sometimes his ailments begin after a vaccination.

Prescribing note: Silicea generally acts very slowly, except in treating splinters.

Keynote Symptoms

- Lacks physical drive
- Low self-esteem
- Easily tired and easily startled
- Poor appetite and poor assimilation of foods

Modalities

Worse: cold; being uncovered; after a vaccination.
Better: being warmly wrapped up; hot applications.

Primary Indicated Conditions

boils	sinusitis
constipation	splinters
diarrhea	

SILICEA

STAPHYSAGRIA
(Common name: Stavesacre)

Overview

Stavesacre is an ancient herb that was used as an emetic (something which causes vomiting) and a cathartic (something which causes evacuation of the bowels). This herb is so poisonous that an externally applied tincture of it was at one time used to kill lice. Its seeds are particularly poisonous. *Staphysagria* is made from these poisonous seeds.

This medicine is very commonly used today because of its special value in treating symptoms that arise from sexual or physical abuse.

Stavesacre is a member of the *Rananculaceae* family like *Aconitum* and *Pulsatilla*.

General Characteristics

Staphysagria is a remedy more commonly given based on the child's emotional state than on a specific physical condition. The exceptions to this general rule are physical injuries such as circumcision, cuts and stabs, insect bites, stings, and surgery incisions.

Staphysagria is a primary remedy for children who suppress their anger and try to firmly control their feelings. This child silently stews about his problems. He can, however, repress his feelings for only so long; eventually he explodes in rage. He trembles, loses his voice, throws things, demands something but then refuses it once it is offered, has great difficulty concentrating, becomes exhausted, and has insomnia. He becomes sensitive to the least offense. Every word said to the child is taken offensively. Once he finally explodes or expresses his anger in some way, he tends to feel remorseful about it. This type of child gets his physical ailments shortly after this suppression of anger or after expressing his rage.

STAPHYSAGRIA

Catherine Coulter, author of *Portraits of Homeopathic Medicines,* describes how a *Staphysagria* child adapts to the offenses he experiences. By "invoking humility to counteract his humiliation, he tries all the harder to placate or ingratiate himself with his offender; in consequence, he is (predictably) forced to put up with even more insult and injury."

This personality trait and response well typifies that of many children who experience sexual or physical abuse. Whether it be because of the abuse or simply because of their own interest, these children tend to dwell on sexual things. As infants and young children, they touch their genitals often, and as they get older, they masturbate frequently.

A child who responds to *Staphysagria* may also become sick after being embarrassed. If, for instance, a younger sibling or friend beats him in a contest, or if he was insulted but was too proud to respond, he may brood about the incident incessantly. When these children swallow their pride, they also suppress their natural self-expression, thus creating an ill state. Embarrassment and then ill health may also be experienced when the child is unable to meet his parents' high expectations.

When the child feels physical pain, it is noticeably worse from touching the painful part. Even the least touch aggravates it.

The child is excessively hungry, even after a meal. He has particular cravings for bread, milk, and fluids.

Staphysagria is a primary remedy for various kinds of puncture wounds: cuts, insect bites and stings, surgery incisions, and circumcision.

Keynote Symptoms

- Ailments after suppressed anger
- Ailments after physical or sexual abuse
- Ailments after embarrassment
- Sensitive to the least touch on the painful part

STAPHYSAGRIA

Modalities

Worse: from anger; embarrassment; pent-up feelings; physical or sexual abuse; least touch or pressure; early morning.
Better: after a meal; when warm; after a night's rest.

Primary Indicated Conditions

anger
bites and stings
circumcision
cuts
cystitis
grief

insomnia
puncture wounds
styes
surgery
toothache

SULPHUR
(Common name: Sulphur)

Overview

Sulphur is an ancient remedy that has been used for thousands of years in a variety of applications treating innumerable complaints. It is externally applied and internally ingested, and people commonly bathe in sulphur springs.

Sulphur is one of the constituents of protoplasm, and as such it has an affinity to every tissue of the body. It can both cause and cure a very wide range of acute and chronic conditions.

When ignited, sulphur burns, creating its distinctive sour, rotten-egg odor. Distinct from phosphorus, which rises and lightens when it is heated, sulphur descends to earth. Perhaps this explains why children who tend to need *Phosphorus* are airy and spacey, while those who need *Sulphur* are down to earth and even dirty.

General Characteristics

Sulphur is a very common remedy for chronic ailments. It is one of the most frequently prescribed of the constitutional medicines (which require professional knowledge to use effectively). It is, however, also effective for certain acute problems. Knowledge about some of the key constitutional characteristics of *Sulphur* children helps us to prescribe this remedy accurately in acute care.

Children helped by *Sulphur* are as active as erupting volcanoes; they create commotions of various sorts. This kind of child tends to be active all the time. He can rarely sit still and can never *stand* still. He is intensely curious and is always investigating things fearlessly. He will climb on trees or furniture to see something that interests him, and when the family is visiting friends, he may wander through the house, yard, or neighborhood, whether he is given permission to do so or not. He also breaks rules, usually because he feels that rules don't apply to him.

The child is a great mess-maker and is careless with others' possessions. He often leaves his clothes and toys strewn all over the house or at a friend's, and will leave the cap off the toothpaste. He is a collector, whether baseball cards or dolls, insects or books. His packrat nature won't let him throw away old or ragged clothes because these clothes have priceless memories attached to them. The child seems to attract dirt and is always dirty. Yet, he never seems to notice or mind it and doesn't like to bathe. And like a volcano, the child has a predeliction to spit.

This kind of child tends to be selfish. He is engrossed in his own world and ignores the needs of others. His selfishness is clear in his attitude toward possessions: In *Portraits of Homeopathic Medicines,* Catherine Coulter describes this attitude as "What's mine is mine, and what's yours is negotiable."

SULPHUR

The child has a natural intelligence that enables him to quickly perceive and integrate new information, and he is a great talker. He loves idiosyncratic facts and figures, and he loves to create his own theories about things, usually speaking with complete authority about them whether he has the authority or not. He loves to think abstractly about things and will ask those impossible-to-answer questions about God, nature, and infinity. He frequently asks "Why?" He also has a tendency to stretch the truth, not to be malicious, but primarily because he gets caught up in his own self-importance and because he likes the attention he gets from telling fantastic stories.

Despite his hyperactivity, the child is also lazy. He does not like doing chores, and he resents his parents or anyone telling him what to do because he feels he could do it better if he was simply left alone. Even if the child promises to do something, he will procrastinate. If given a choice, the child would sleep late, hang out in his bedroom playing games, and frequently sneak into the kitchen for snacks.

Also like a volcano, these children are hot and are aggravated by heat. Their symptoms are made worse from warm weather, warmth of a bed, warm rooms, and warm clothing (especially wool). Whether the child has a fever or not, he does not like to wear much clothing. His feet become particularly hot at night, and he either sticks them out of the bed or throws off all the covers. He likes cool temperatures but can be aggravated by exposure to extreme cold.

The child's heated state shows itself in a reddened face and reddened mucous membranes, including red lips, red margins of eyelids, nostrils, and ears.

To generate and maintain all this heat and activity, this kind of child has a large appetite, except for breakfast. He craves salt, fats, spicy foods (pizza is one of his favorites), and especially sweets (chocolate and ice cream in particular). Unlike most children, this child will eat unusual foods which the

SULPHUR

average child will avoid. True to his messy nature, he often eats with his fingers. He is very thirsty, especially for ice-cold sodas. He usually dislikes milk, and if he does drink it, he will sometimes become extremely irritable or experience digestive problems, diarrhea, or headaches.

The child has dirty-looking, dry, rough skin. Despite this fact, he has an aversion to water and bathing. He also has offensive body odors and discharges.

Sulphur is known to be one of the most helpful homeopathic medicines for treating acute conditions that linger, such as colds, flus, coughs, and ear infections.

Keynote Symptoms

- Physically hot but aggravated by heat or anything warm
- Reddened mucous membranes, especially the lips
- Messy children with dry, dirty-looking skin

Modalities

Worse: heat; warm room; warmth of bed; extreme cold; standing; bathing.
Better: in the open air; cool air; scratching.

Primary Indicated Conditions

allergies	impetigo
bedwetting	measles
boils	poison ivy or oak
fever	sore throat
headaches	styes
hives	

SULPHUR

SYMPHYTUM
(Common name: Comfrey)

Overview

The word *Symphytum* is taken from the Greek word *symphyo,* which means "to unite." The common name of this herb, comfrey, is adapted from the words *con firma,* which alludes to the uniting of bones, a healing action which people for several centuries have observed from using this herb. In fact, other names for comfrey in folklore are knitbone and boneset.

Comfrey is rich in calcium, phosphorus, potassium, iron, and magnesium, as well as vitamins B, C, and E. Looking at the law of similars, one might wonder how and why an herb that is rich in calcium would be useful in homeopathic dosages for people with fractures. Calcium is indeed valuable for building strong bones; however, because overdoses of calcium actually cause brittle bones, homeopathic doses of calcium can help to strengthen them.

Comfrey also contains a chemical called allantoin which has been found to promote the growth of new cells. In fact, numerous over-the-counter and prescription skin creams contain this valuable healing substance.

General Characteristics

Symphytum is the primary remedy for fractures. If a child has a fracture that is healing slowly, *Symphytum* or *Calcarea phosphorica* should be considered. It is also a remedy for injury to the periosteum.

Symphytum is a very effective remedy for a child who is hit with a blunt instrument which creates black and blue bruises. Typically, *Symphytum* is indicated primarily when this injury does not actually break the skin.

A child usually gets a black eye when he gets hit there. *Symphytum* is a valuable remedy for these injuries, whether the tissue around the eye is injured or the eyeball itself is affected. (Medical care should also be sought if the latter is the case.)

Keynote Symptoms

- Bruises from blunt instruments
- Black eye or black and blue marks from injury
- Injury to the periosteum (the bone covering)
- Fractures

Primary Indicated Conditions

bruises   fracture
eye injuries

SYMPHYTUM

PART 5

Commercial Homeopathic Medicines

~

COMBINATION MEDICINES

Since the early days of homeopathy, homeopaths have combined two or more homeopathic medicines in the belief that one of the ingredients or the resulting mixture may heal a particular ailment. Some advocates of homeopathy consider such mixtures to be blasphemy, since one of homeopathy's basic principles is to individualize a medicine to a person's unique symptoms. However, people continue to use these combination formulas because they do work.

Many members of the public may, in fact, be more familiar with these homeopathic combination medicines than they are with individual homeopathic medicines since these formulas are marketed more aggressively. Combination medicines are very popular in Europe, especially Germany, and they are quite popular among consumers in the United States as well.

Typically, three to eight homeopathic medicines are mixed together to create a combination medicine. The ingredients usually consist of low-potency medicines (below the 24x potency) which are particularly effective in treating a specific condition. For example, five of the most common remedies for hay fever may be combined to treat a broader spectrum of persons suffering from this condition. These user-friendly homeopathic medicines are easier to prescribe than a single homeopathic medicine since you don't have to individualize a specific remedy to a person's unique set of symptoms. Also, just as many herbalists recommend a specific combination of herbs for their ability to act synergistically, a good homeopathic combination medicine may sometimes be more effective in acute disorders because of its synergistic effect.

Dr. Steven Subotnick, podiatric physician and surgeon and author of numerous books on sports medicine, including *Sports and Exercise Injuries: Conventional, Homeopathic, and Alternative Treatments,* uses homeopathic medicines to treat a wide variety of foot problems and to help speed healing after foot surgery. Because of the frequency with which he performs foot surgery, Dr. Subotnick has had the opportunity to closely observe the benefits of individual homeopathic medicines as compared to mixtures of homeopathic medicines.

Dr. Subotnick has found that *Arnica* is helpful, but that it is even more effective when he also gives *Hypericum* and *Ruta*. He asserts, "*Arnica* helps the patient deal with the shock of surgery and speeds the healing of soft tissues, while *Hypericum* helps to heal the nerves, and *Ruta* works to heal trauma to the bone. Together they work much better than when I use them individually." Dr. Subotnick makes up his own homeopathic combination medicines, though he also uses a commercial homeopathic product that includes these three medicines and others.

Dr. Joe D. Goldstrich, a homeopath and cardiologist who practices in Dallas, Texas, had this to say about combination medicines:

> As a classical homeopathic physician, I previously looked down on combination remedies. As my practice grew, I saw how much time I was spending prescribing for colds and flu. Even when I got the correct remedy on the first prescription, the symptoms would change in a few days, usually necessitating a change to a new remedy and even more time going over new symptoms. I tried a combination medicine for colds and flu (Longevity's) on myself when I got the flu. The

results were amazing—I was well in 36 hours. I next tried it with my son. Same results. Next I gave it to another son and told him to take a dose at the first sign of a cold. He aborted the whole thing with *one dose!* Many of my patients keep combination remedies at home so they can begin taking them at the first sign of this condition. It really works, and it makes my work a lot easier.

But some advocates of homeopathy do not consider combination medicines to be true homeopathy. They assert that using these combination medicines makes it impossible to know which individual homeopathic ingredient was the most effective. Moreover, these combination medicines tend to only temporarily relieve chronic symptoms, rarely curing them. For instance, a child who is given a combination medicine for chronically recurring hay fever may have his symptoms temporarily relieved, but usually the hay fever symptoms will eventually return. The underlying allergy to pollen has not been cured. However, this is also true about many of the individual homeopathic medicines described in this book. The successful cure of *chronic* symptoms usually requires the skill of a professional homeopath who has a broad range of knowledge of the individual homeopathic medicines, who uses an effective sequence of remedies on follow-up visits, and who knows when to stop giving remedies as improvement begins to take place.

Despite the value and the ease of taking combination medicines, the power of an individually chosen, single homeopathic medicine should not be underestimated. A correctly chosen homeopathic medicine can deeply heal a chronic or even hereditary condition and raise an individual's overall level of health, making him more resistant to both physical and psychological stress.

If, however, your child has chronic symptoms and you do not have access to a professional homeopath, if you cannot determine which individual homeopathic medicine to give, or if what seems to be the correct medicine isn't working or isn't immediately available to you, combination medicines can often provide relief. And because combination medicines are considerably safer than using conventional drugs, these remedies have an important place in your home medicine kit.

It's easy to pick a combination medicine for your child's acute complaint. The medicines are clearly labeled for various conditions; for example, teething, colic, allergies, headache. However, because the formula in a combination medicine will vary from one manufacturer to the next, it can be difficult to determine which brand might be most effective. There are, however, a few guidelines to follow.

First, use medicines from a reputable manufacturer (such companies are listed in the Resources section of this book), or a formula created by a known and respected homeopath. Second, your own experience with the combination medicine or knowledge of each homeopathic ingredient in the formula gives further support for its value. Finally, certain homeopathic texts (notably Kent's *Repertory* and Boericke's *Pocket Manual of Materia Medica with Repertory*, the B. Jain edition) provide information about how certain homeopathic ingredients interact with each other. It makes sense to use a combination medicine that does not contain ingredients that are either known to counteract each other or that interact poorly together. (Medicines listed in the above-mentioned books as *inimical* to each other suggests that the medicines not be given together or in sequence.)

Homeopathic combination medicines do indeed have a place in your medicine cabinet. They are easy to prescribe, are often effective, and are generally more accessible through health food stores and pharmacies than the individual remedies. Ultimately, however, it is generally agreed that an individually chosen homeopathic medicine will act faster, longer, and deeper than the combination formula. By recognizing the value of individual medicines and the combination formulas, you can benefit from both of them.

EXTERNAL APPLICATIONS

Most homeopathic remedies are medicines taken internally. Even skin diseases are treated internally because homeopaths assume that symptoms of skin disease represent an internal disorder that is simply revealing itself on the skin.

There are, however, good reasons to use external homeopathic applications, such as for healing injuries and chafings, bites and stings, and various kinds of burns. These medicines can augment the body's healing powers and prevent potential complications. External applications are not significantly diluted or potentized like other homeopathic medicines. Because these applications are of herbal origin, they can be considered either homeopathic or herbal medicines (though homeopaths will sometimes use them for different symptoms and for different reasons than herbalists).

There are several kinds of external applications, including tinctures, low-alcohol solutions, nonalcoholic solutions, ointments, creams, gels, oils, lotions, and sprays. Each external application has its benefits and limitations.

It is generally best to apply these external applications with a clean cotton swab. Avoid dipping a cotton swab back into a bottle after you have wiped a wound; you may accidentally transfer bacteria from the wound to the bottle. You can also use your fingers to apply external applications, though it is not recommended for treating deep cuts or severe burns. If, however, you do use your fingers, wash them first.

Because homeopathic external applications are not potentized, they are not sensitive to being antidoted by the various substances discussed in part 2, nor is it necessary to follow the normal precautions, such as avoiding food and drink for fifteen minutes before and after using the medicine.

Like many conventional medical external applications, many of the following homeopathic external applications include ingredients which are inappropriate for internal consumption and may even be dangerous. You should make sure that these medicines are stored away from the reach of babies and young children.

Tinctures

A tincture is generally a high-alcohol solution, usually 35–90 percent alcohol. *Arnica* and *Calendula* tincture both are 45 percent alcohol, while *Hypericum* is 65 percent alcohol.

Tinctures are an extract of an herb in an alcohol base. Alcohol is used both to extract constituents from an herb and to preserve the solution. Because alcohol itself has antiseptic properties, a tincture helps fight and prevent infection. It is best to use a tincture on open wounds because of its antiseptic properties. A tincture also allows the skin to breathe, which keeps the wound from becoming too moist, thus preventing it from becoming a breeding ground for further infection.

Dilute tinctures slightly before applying them to a wound (one part tincture to three or four parts water); their high alcohol solution can cause burning and stinging. *For deep wounds, it is safest to dilute a tincture either with freshly boiled water or filtered, sterilized water (available in many pharmacies).* Generally, tap or bottled water is adequate for most common cuts or burns. Although tinctures allow the wounded skin to breathe, they also tend to dry out the skin due to the high alcohol content. Prevent this problem by not using the tincture too frequently or by alternating the use of a tincture with that of an ointment, spray, cream, gel, or oil.

One other problem with tinctures is that they are easily washed off, either by water or sweat.

The tinctures of many homeopathic single remedies are

available through homeopathic manufacturers, though those substances that are potentially toxic when used internally in tincture form are only available by prescription from a medical doctor.

Low-Alcohol Solutions

A homeopathic low-alcohol solution, generally called a *succus,* contains 15–20 percent alcohol. The benefits of this application is that it can be applied directly to shallow wounds, chafings, or burns. A succus does not dry out the skin as much as a tincture, so it can be used more frequently.

Homeopathic companies generally make low-alcohol solutions of a limited number of medicines, usually *Arnica, Calendula, Hypericum,* and *Apis.*

Most of the other external applications are not made with alcohol, though they are made with some type of petroleum product or vegetable oil.

Non-Alcohol Solutions

Non-alcohol solutions can be applied directly to an injured area without being diluted with water and create minimal stinging upon application to a wound. Unlike tinctures, which can dry the skin too much, non-alcohol solutions tend to moisturize the skin, though in doing so, they sometimes inhibit the skin from breathing.

Some companies offer a non-alcohol *Calendula* solution made with water and vegetable glycerin (usually derived from coconut oil). This solution contains 22 percent *Calendula* extractables, which is almost twice as concentrated as it is in the tincture or succus. It is not, however, as well preserved as a tincture, and if it is not completely used within a year it will lose its potency. It should be kept in a cool, dry place or perhaps refrigerated after opening if you don't think you'll finish it in a year (this refrigeration should not be colder than 40 degrees Fahrenheit).

Homeopathic companies generally make only a limited number of non-alcohol solutions, usually *Arnica* and *Calendula.*

Ointments

Ointments are generally made with petrolatum, which is a purified rock oil taken from the earth and is considered a petroleum derivative. This oil helps moisturize the skin and does not wash off easily, thus making it useful when it is applied to a wound or burn on the hands or any part frequently used or exposed to water. Ointments also help moisturize the skin. They are easy to apply and reapply when the dressing needs to be changed.

Don't use an ointment on an open wound or deep cut; it will lead to increased moisture and create a breeding ground for infection. You can consider using an ointment on superficial wounds or on a wound that is almost healed.

Sometimes an ointment is used on skin inflammations such as eczema or herpes. Although these applications will not cure the condition, they often provide soothing temporary relief.

Homeopathic companies usually make ointments of *Aesculus, Apis, Arnica, Calendula, Graphites, Hamamelis, Hippozaenium, Hypericum, Ledum, Symphytum, Thuja, Urtica urens,* and some combination remedies for hemorrhoids or warts.

Creams

A cream can be variable in its contents. It generally consists of two basic parts: one part is oily or greasy and the other is watery. The oily part is commonly made from petrolatum (the same ingredient in Vaseline), lanolin (from lamb's wool), beeswax or paraffin (creating a thicker cream), or stearic acid (a fatty acid). The watery part can be made from aloe vera, glycerin (a clear syrupy liquid made from vegetable or animal fat), or simply water.

The benefit of a cream is that it moisturizes the skin, and it is not as heavy as an ointment, thus allowing the skin to breathe more easily. It is best to use creams when the skin around a wound is very dry or when an external application needs to be used frequently. Because cream tends to wash off more quickly than ointments or oils, you may need to apply it more often if the wound is washed or wiped.

Homeopathic companies generally make creams of a limited number of medicines, usually *Arnica, Calendula,* and *Urtica urens.*

Gels

Gels provide a cool feeling to a wound or burn. They can be applied directly to the injury, though there may be a slight stinging sensation on some wounds. The gels are usually very easy to spread onto the skin, and a little bit tends to go a long way. Gels leave a less greasy residue and because of this are more easily washed off.

Gels tend to dry the skin in a wound or around the wound. If the skin gets too dry, use a cream or ointment.

Gels, like oils, are also particularly good for animals with fur because the gel is able to penetrate the fur to the skin.

Most homeopathic companies make gels for only a limited number of medicines, usually *Arnica, Calendula,* and combinations for bites and stings.

Oils

Oils are usually made with mineral oil (a petroleum-based product), though they are sometimes made with vegetable oils. They can be applied directly to a wound and don't sting.

They moisturize the skin, though they do not allow the skin to breathe well, so they should not be used on deep wounds or serious burns. They do not wash off easily, making them good for someone who washes or swims frequently or who often uses the part of his body that is wounded.

Many massage practitioners use *Arnica* oil as a massage lotion.

Medicated oils should not be confused with essential oils, which are naturally occurring oils that are extracted directly from botanical materials.

Lotions

A lotion is a thin cream or liquid. It tends to be less thick than a cream or ointment and more thick than a tincture or an oil. Lotions are usually not too greasy, can be easily washed off, and are easily applied and spread.

Some lotions have supplements in them to moisturize the skin, such as aloe vera, avocado oil, or apricot kernel oil. To give the lotion consistency the manufacturer usually adds emulsifiers, which may be from a natural or synthetic source.

Other kinds of lotions have a liquid consistency because they are a mixture of a tincture and isopropyl alcohol. These lotions can be applied directly to a wound. They dry immediately and leave no greasy feeling. They may cause some slight stinging pain upon application.

There are only three common homeopathic lotions: *Arnica, Calendula,* and *Hypericum.*

Sprays

Applying external homeopathic medicines from a spray bottle is a new and useful development. Spray bottles provide convenience because the parent or even the child can simply spray the affected part. Spray bottles also tend to be more hygienic than other applications because cotton swabs are not required. (When using other types of external applications, you can sometimes touch the lip of the bottle with the cotton swab, picking up germs accidentally placed there by a previous cotton swab.)

The ingredients in the spray bottles are usually an herbal extract with glycerine and water or an herbal tincture with isopropyl alcohol. Because products made with glycerine and water do not contain alcohol as a preservative, it is recommended that they be kept in a cold place, ideally in a refrigerator.

Products made with isopropyl alcohol will burn slightly when sprayed on an open wound. These products will tend to dry out the skin when used frequently. They also tend to wash off easily. If it is necessary to frequently re-apply a product to a cut or burn, consider alternating a spray with an ointment, lotion, or oil, which helps provide moisture to the skin. Finally, since the sprays generally contain isopropyl alcohol, make sure a child does not accidentally ingest them.

APPENDIX I

Homeopathic Research

If you've purchased this book you probably do not need to be convinced about the value of homeopathic medicines. However, a spouse, parent, relative, neighbor, or doctor is often skeptical about this unique type of medicine. It may be helpful, then, to at least describe briefly some of the research that has been published about the use of homeopathic medicines. Readers interested in more information about research on homeopathy are recommended to read my earlier book, *Discovering Homeopathy.*[1]

There are actually many more published studies on homeopathy than most people realize. The *British Medical Journal* published a review of twenty-five years of clinical research on homeopathy.[2] The researchers described 107 controlled clinical trials, 81 of which showed successful results from the homeopathic medicines. Of these 107 studies, a significant percentage of the highest-quality experiments showed positive results from homeopathic medicines.

Of the studies reviewed, 13 of the 19 trials showed successful treatment of respiratory infections, 6 of 7 trials showed positive results in treating other infections, 5 of 7 showed improvement in diseases of the digestive system, 5 of 5 showed successful treatment of hay fever, 5 of 7 showed faster recovery after abdominal surgery, 4 of 6 promoted healing in treating rheumatological disease, 18 of 20 showed benefit in addressing pain or trauma, 8 of 10 showed positive results in relieving mental or psychological problems, and 13 of 15 showed improvement from various diagnoses.

Of special interest to mothers-to-be, research has indicated that homeopathic medicines can reduce the time of labor and the complications from birth.[3] Ninety women in their
last month of pregnancy were tested with a combination of
five homeopathic medicines (*Caulophylllum, Arnica, Pulsatilla, Gelsemium,* and *Cimicifuga*) given in the 5c potency. The
women given this mixture of homeopathic medicines spent
40 percent less time in labor and had approximately one-
quarter as many complications during birth as compared to
the women given a placebo.

A study of hay fever, which compared patients given a
homeopathic medicine with those given a placebo, allowed
patients to use an antihistamine if the tested medicine was
not working adequately.[4] The remedy used was a mixture of
twelve different pollens in the 30c potency. The research,
which was published in *The Lancet,* showed that those given a
placebo felt the need to take the antihistamine twice as often
as those given the homeopathic medicine.

A study of 487 patients with influenza showed that a
homeopathic medicine, *Anas barbariae* 200c, was effective;
almost twice as many patients given this remedy had their flu
symptoms completely resolved within 48 hours, as compared
with the patients given a placebo.[5] This study was published in
the *British Journal of Clinical Pharmacology* and received special commendation from the *The Lancet.*[6]

One study soon to be published conducted at a University
of Glasgow hospital showed that homeopathic medicines can
successfully treat asthma. Considering the seriousness of this
condition, the increasing numbers of children who are actually dying from it, and the potential dangers of some of the
conventional drugs used to treat it, it is worthwhile to know
that homeopathic medicines offer a safe and often effective alternative to conventional therapies.

That homeopathic medicines have not been tested for
every common ailment is to be expected, given the limited research funds available for homeopathic research. But even if

there has not yet been formal research on the specific ailment your child is suffering from, this doesn't mean that homeopathic medicines are ineffective in dealing with it. It simply means that no standard research study has yet examined it.

However, you can be certain that homeopathic physicians have successfully treated virtually every common health condition of children. This doesn't mean that homeopathic medicines can cure every child. It does, however, mean that homeopathic medicines can, when correctly prescribed, at least significantly improve the health of a child and do so without side effects.

In addition to the various clinical studies using homeopathic medicines, there have been numerous laboratory experiments. There has, for instance, been research that has shown that homeopathic medicines stimulate the immune system's macrophages[7] (a large cell that devours potential disease-causing microorganisms and foreign particles), that eight out of ten specific homeopathic remedies tested had antiviral action,[8] and that homeopathic microdoses of arsenic stimulated the ability of rats to excrete poisonous doses of arsenic.[9]

There have also been several studies that have shown that homeopathic medicines are *not* effective; however, each of these studies contained significant flaws in design. These studies simply tested a single homeopathic medicine in its effectiveness in treating a specific condition. Although homeopaths have found that certain remedies can be effective in treating specific conditions, most of the time it is essential to individualize a remedy to the person based on matching patterns of symptoms.

Despite the various studies showing the value of the homeopathic medicines, there is a real need for more research. Sadly, the American government and most other governments have never funded homeopathic research. Also, no major medical or scientific philanthropic organizations have funded investigations on homeopathic medicine. Hopefully, as more people obtain benefits from homeopathic medicines, public and private funds will finally be devoted to investigating this important area of medicine.

References

[1] Dana Ullman. *Discovering Homeopathy: Medicine for the 21st Century.* Berkeley: North Atlantic, 1991.

[2] J. Kleijnen, P. Knipschild, and Gerben ter Riet. "Clinical Trials of Homeopathy." *British Medical Journal* 302 (February 9, 1991): 316–323.

[3] P. Dorfman, M. Lasserre, M. Tetau. "Preparation a' l'accouchement par homeopathie: Experimentation en double-insu versus placebo" [Preparation for Birth by Homeopathy: Experimentation by Double-blind Placebo]. *Cahiers de Biotherapie* 94 (April 1987): 77–81.

[4] David Taylor Reilly, Morag A. Taylor, Charles McSharry, and Tom Aitchison. "Is Homeopathy a Placebo Response: Controlled Trial of Homeopathic Potency, with Pollen in Hayfever as Model." *Lancet* (October 18, 1986): 881–886.

[5] J. P. Zmirou, D. D'Adhemar, D. and F. Balducci. "A Controlled Evaluation of a Homeopathic Preparation in the Treatment of Influenza-like Syndromes." *British Journal of Clinical Pharmacology* 299 (1989): 365–366.

[6] "Quadruple Blind," *Lancet* (April 4, 1989): 91.

[7] Elizabeth Davenas, Bernard Poitevin, and Jacques Benveniste. "Effect on Mouse Peritoneal Macrophages of Orally Administered Very High Dilutions of Silica." *European Journal of Pharmacology* 135 (April 1987): 313–319.

[8] L. M. Singh and G. Gupta. "Antiviral Efficacy of Homeopathic Drugs Against Animal Viruses." *British Homeopathic Journal* 74 (July 1985): 168–174.

[9] J. C. Cazin et al. "A Study of the Effect of Decimal and Centesimal Dilution of Arsenic on Retention and Mobilization of Arsenic in the Rat." *Human Toxicology* (July 1987): 315–320.

APPENDIX II

Homeopathic Medicines and Their Pronunciations

Medicines with an asterisk are recommended as an integral part of your home medicine kit.

Aconitum* [ak-ō-nīt'-um] (monkshood)

Aethusa [e-thoo'-za] (fool's parsley)

Allium cepa* [al'-lē-um sē'-pa] (onion)

Alumina [a-loo'-me-na] (aluminum)

Ambrosia [am-brō'-zha] (ragweed)

Anas barbariae* [an-as bar-bar'-ē-a] (heart and liver of a duck) (marketed as Oscillococcinum* [os-sēl'-lō-ko-sī'-num])

Antimonium crudum [an-ti-mō'-nē-um krood'-um] (black sulphide of antimony)

Antimonium tartaricum [an-ti-mō'-nē-um tar-tar'-i-kum] (tartar emetic)

Apis* [ā'-pis] (crushed bee)

Argentum nitricum [ar-jen'-tum nī'-tri-kum] (silver nitrate)

Arnica* (in potency, gel, spray, oil, and ointment) [ar'-ne-ka] (mountain daisy)

Arsenicum album* [ar-sen'-i-kum al'-bum] (white arsenic)

Belladonna* [bel-a-don'-a] (deadly nightshade)

Bellis perennis [bel'-lis pe-ren'-niss] (daisy)

Borax [bōr'-aks] (borate of sodium)

Bryonia* [brī-ō'-nē-a] (wild hops)

Calcarea carbonica* [kal-ka'-rē-a kar-bon'-i-ka] (carbonate of lime)

Calcarea phosphorica [kal-ka' rē-a fos-for'-i-ka] (phosphate of lime)

Calendula* (tincture, lotion, spray, gel, and ointment) [ka'-len-du-la] (marigolds)

Cantharis* [kan'-thar-is] (spanish fly)

Causticum [kaus'-ti-kum] (potassium hydrate)

Chamomilla* [kam-ō-mil'-la] (chamomille)

Chelidonium [chel-i-dō'-nē-um] (great celandine)

Cinchona [sin-khō'-na] (Peruvian bark)

Cocculus [kok'-ū-lus] (Indian cockle)

Coffea cruda [kof'-fe-a kroo'-da] (coffee)

Colocynthis* [kol'-ō-sin'-this] (bitter cucumber)

Croton tiglium [krō'-ton tig'-lē-um] (croton oil seed)

Cuprum [koo'-prum] (copper)

Drosera [drō'-zhe-ra] (sundew)

Equisetum [ek-we-sē'-tum] (horsetail)

Eupatorium perfoliatum [ū-pa-to'-rē-um per-fō-le-a'-tum] (boneset)

Euphrasia* [ū-frā'-zha] (eyebright)

Ferrum phosphoricum* (fer'-rum fos-for'-i-kum] (phosphate of iron)

Gelsemium* [jel-se'-mē-um] (yellow jasmine)

Glonoine [glon'-o-ēn] (nitroglycerine)

Graphites [gra-fī'-teez] (black lead)

Hepar sulphur* [hē'-par sul'-fur] (calcium sulphide)

Hydrastis [hī-dras'-tis] (golden seal)

Hypericum* (in potency and tincture) [hī-per'-i-kum] (St. John's wort)

Ignatia* [ig-nā'-sha] (St. Ignatius bean)

Influenzinum [in-flu-en-zi'-num] (influenza virus)

Ipecacuahna* [ip-e-kak'-ū-an-nya'] (ipecac root)

Iris [ī'-ris] (blue flag)

Kali bichromicum* [ka'-lē bī' chrō' -me-kum] (bichromate of potash)

Kreosotum [krē-ō-sō'-tum] (beechwood kreosote)

Lachesis [lak'-e-sis] (venom of the bushmaster)

Ledum* [lē'-dum] (wild rosemary)

Lobelia [lō-bē'-lē-a] (Indian tobacco)

Lycopodium [lī-kō-pō'-dē-um] (club moss)

Magnesia phosphoricum* [mag-nē'-zhē-a fos-for'-i-cum] (phosphate of magnesia)

Mercurius* [mer-cu'-rē-us] (mercury)

Natrum muriaticum [na'-trum mu-rē-at'-i-kum] (sodium chloride/salt)

Natrum sulphuricum [na'-trum sul-fur'-i-kum] (sulphate of sodium)

Nux vomica* [nux vom'-i-ka] (poison nut)

Petroleum [pe-trō'-lē-um] (crude rock oil)

Phosphorus* [fos'-for-us] (phosphorus)

Phytolacca [fī-tō-lak'-ka] (pokeroot)

Pilocarpinum [pi-lō-kar-pī'-num] (pilocarpinum)

Plantago [plan-tā'-gō] (plantain)

Podophyllum* [pōd-ō-fī'-lum] (may apple)

Pulsatilla* [pul-sa-til'-la] (windflower)

Rhus toxicodendron* [rus tox-i-kō-den'-dron] (poison ivy)

Ruta* (roo'-ta) (rue)

Sabadilla [sa-ba-dil'-la] (cevadilla seed)

Sambucus [sam-bū'-kus] (elder)

Sanguinaria [san-gwi-na'-rē-a] (bloodroot)

Sarsaparilla [sar-sa-pa-ril'-la] (smilax)

Sepia [sē'-pe-a] (cuttlefish)

Silicea* [si-lē'-sē-a] (silica)

Spigelia [spi-je'-lē-a] (pinkroot)

Spongia [spun'-jē-a] (roasted sponge)

Staphysagria* [staf-i-sa'-grē-a] (stavesacre)

Sulphur* [sul'-fur] (sulphur)

Symphytum* [sim-fī'-tum] (comfrey)

Tabacum [ta-bak'-um] (tobacco)

Urtica urens [ur-ti'-ka u'-rens] (stinging nettle)

Veratrum album [ve-ra'-trum al'-bum] (white hellebore)

Wyethia [why-ē'-thē-a] (poison weed)

Resources

RECOMMENDED READING

Introductory and Family Care Books

The following books provide general information about homeopathy and homeopathic medicines. Although most of these books are not written primarily about treating children, they each contain information useful for their treatment.

Buegel, Dale, Blair Lewis, and Dennis Chernin. *Homeopathic Remedies for Health Professionals and Laypeople.* Revised. Honesdale, PA: Himalayan, 1991.

Castro, Miranda. *The Complete Homeopathy Handbook.* New York: St. Martin's, 1991.

Cummings, Stephen, and Dana Ullman. *Everybody's Guide to Homeopathic Medicines.* Revised and expanded. Los Angeles: Jeremy Tarcher, 1991.

Kruzel, Thomas. *The Homeopathic Emergency Handbook.* Berkeley: North Atlantic, 1992.

Lockie, Andrew. *The Family Guide to Homeopathy.* New York: Prentice-Hall, 1991.

Moskowitz, Richard. *Homeopathic Medicines for Pregnancy and Childbirth.* Berkeley: North Atlantic, 1992.

Panos, Maesimund, and Jane Heimlich. *Homeopathic Medicine at Home.* Los Angeles: Jeremy Tarcher, 1980.

Smith, Trevor. *Homeopathic Medicines for Women.* Rochester, VT: Healing Arts, 1989.

Ullman, Dana. *Discovering Homeopathy: Medicine for the 21st Century.* Berkeley: North Atlantic, 1991.

Vithoulkas, George. *Homeopathy: Medicine for the New Man.* New York: Arco, 1979.

Philosophy, Methodology, and Research

These books describe homeopathic philosophy so that you can better understand this unique medical system. They also provide instruction on the homeopathic approach to healing.

Coulter, Harris L. *Homeopathic Science and Modern Medicine: The Physics of Healing with Microdoses.* Berkeley: North Atlantic, 1981.

Dhawale, M. L. *Principles and Practice of Homeopathy.* Bombay: D. K. Homeopathic Corporation, 1967.

Hahnemann, Samuel. *Organon of Medicine.* Reprint. New Delhi: B. Jain.

Kent, James Tyler. *Lectures on Homeopathic Philosophy.* Reprint. Berkeley: North Atlantic, 1979.

Koehler, Gerhard. *The Handbook of Homeopathy.* Rochester, VT: Healing Arts, 1987.

Roberts, H. A. *The Principles and Art of Cure by Homoeopathy.* Reprint. New Delhi: B. Jain.

Vithoulkas, George. *The Science of Homeopathy.* New York: Grove, 1979.

Wright, Elizabeth Hubbard. *A Brief Study Course in Homeopathy.* St. Louis: Formur, 1977.

Materia Medicas and Repertories

These books are at an intermediate and advanced level. They describe the precise symptoms each homeopathic medicine is known to treat. These books will help you prescribe homeopathic medicine more accurately.

Allen, H. C. *Keynotes and Characteristic of the Materia Medica.* Reprint. New Delhi: B. Jain.

Boericke, William. *Pocket Manual of Materia Medica with Repertory.* Reprint. Santa Rosa, CA: Boericke and Tafel.

Clarke, John. *Dictionary of Practical Materia Medica* (3 volumes). Reprint. New Delhi: B. Jain.

Coulter, Catherine. *Portraits of Homeopathic Medicines.* 2 vols. Berkeley: North Atlantic, 1986–1988.

Gibson, D. M. *Studies of Homoeopathic Remedies.* Beaconsfield, England: Beaconsfield Publishers, 1987.

Herscu, Paul. *The Homeopathic Treatment of Children: Pediatric Constitutional Types.* Berkeley: North Atlantic, 1991.

Kent, James Tyler. *Lectures on Homoeopathic Materia Medica.* Reprint. New Delhi: B. Jain.

_____. *Repertory of Homoeopathic Materia Medica.* Reprint. New Delhi: B. Jain.

Nash, E. B. *Leaders in Homoeopathic Therapeutics.* Reprint. New Delhi: B. Jain.

Tyler, Margaret. *Drug Pictures.* Essex, England: C. W. Daniel, 1952.

Wheeler, Charles. *An Introduction to the Principles and Practice of Homoeopathy.* Reprint. New Delhi: B. Jain.

Whitmont, Edward C. *Psyche and Substance: Essays on Homeopathy in the Light of Jungian Psychology.* Berkeley: North Atlantic, 1991.

Source of Homeopathic Books

Homeopathic Educational Services, 2124 Kittredge St., Berkeley, CA 94704

Homeopathic Educational Services is the most comprehensive source of homeopathic books, tapes, medicines, software, and general information in the United States.

Conventional Pediatrics

Berberich, Ralph, and Ann Parker. *The Available Pediatrician: Every Parent's Guide to Common Childhood Illness.* New York: Pantheon, 1988.

Eisenberg, Arlene, Heidi E. Merkoff, and Sandee E. Hathaway. *What to Expect the First Year.* New York: Workman, 1989.

Griffith, H. Winter. *Complete Guide to Pediatric Symptoms, Illnesses, and Medications.* Los Angeles: The Body Press, 1989.

Leach, Penelope. *Your Baby and Child.* Revised. New York: Knopf, 1990.

Pantell, Robert, James F. Fries, and Donald M. Vickery. *Taking Care of Your Child.* Revised. Reading, MA: Addison Wesley, 1990.

Shelov, Steven P., ed. *Care for Your Baby and Your Child (Birth to Age 5).* New York: Bantam, 1991.

Spock, Benjamin, and Michael Rothenberg. *Dr. Spock's Baby and Child Care*. New York: Pocket, 1985.

Natural Health Care for Children

Duncan, Alice L. *Your Health Child*. Los Angeles: Jeremy Tarcher, 1991.

Gardner, Joy. *Healing the Family*. New York: Bantam, 1982.

Neustaedter, Randall. *The Immunization Decision: A Guide for Parents*. Berkeley: North Atlantic, 1990.

Riggs, Maribeth. *Natural Health Care*. New York: Crown, 1989.

Samuels, Michael, and Nancy Samuels. *The Well Child Book*. New York: Summit, 1983.

_____. *The Well Baby Book*. Revised. New York: Summit, 1991.

Schmidt, Michael. *Childhood Ear Infections: What Every Parent and Physician Should Know about Prevention, Home Care, and Alternative Treatment*. Berkeley: North Atlantic, 1990.

Schoenaker, Joyce M., and Charity Y. Vitale. *Healthy Homes, Healthy Kids*. Washington, D.C.: 1991.

Stanway, Andrew. *The Natural Family Doctor*. New York: Fireside, 1987.

Subotnick, Steven. *Sports and Exercise Injuries: Conventional, Homeopathic, and Alternative Treatments*. Berkeley: North Atlantic, 1991.

HOMEOPATHIC MANUFACTURERS

Many of the homeopathic manufacturers also sell homeopathic books.

Biological Homeopathic Industries, 11600 Cochiti S.E., Albuquerque, NM 87123

Boericke and Tafel, 2381 Circadian Way, Santa Rosa, CA 95407

Boiron, 1208 Amosland Road, Norwood, PA 19074. Also: 98c West Cochran, Simi Valley, CA 93065

Dolisos, 3014 Rigel, Las Vegas, NV 89102

Longevity Pure Medicines, 9595 Wilshire Blvd. #706, Beverly Hills, CA 90212

Luyties Pharmacal, 4200 Laclede Ave., St. Louis, MO 63108

Medicine from Nature/Nature's Way, 10 Mountain Springs Road, Springville, UT 84663

Standard Homeopathic Company, 204-210 W. 131st St., Los Angeles, CA 90061

HOMEOPATHIC ORGANIZATIONS

American Association of Homeopathic Pharmacists, P.O. Box 2273, Falls Church, VA 22042

American Institute of Homeopathy, 1585 Glencoe St. #44, Denver, CO 80220

British Homeopathic Association, The Royal London Homeopathic Hospital, Great Ormond St., London WC1N 3HR, England

Foundation for Homeopathic Education and Research, 2124 Kittredge St., Berkeley, CA 94704

International Foundation for Homeopathy, 2366 Eastlake Ave. E. #301, Seattle, WA 98102

National Center for Homeopathy, 801 N. Fairfax #306, Alexandria, VA 22314

The Society of Homoeopaths, 2 Artizan Road, Northampton NN1 4HU, England

HOMEOPATHIC STUDY GROUPS

There are over one hundred and fifty homeopathic study groups throughout the United States where people get together once a week or once a month to learn about homeopathy. The groups are coordinated by the National Center for Homeopathy (see address above). A directory of these groups is available for purchase from the National Center for Homeopathy and from Homeopathic Educational Services.

HOMEOPATHIC SCHOOLS AND TRAINING PROGRAMS IN NORTH AMERICA

Hahnemann College of Homeopathy, 828 San Pablo Ave., Albany, CA 94706

International Foundation for Homeopathy, 2366 Eastlake Ave. E. #301, Seattle, WA 98102

National Center for Homeopathy, 801 N. Fairfax #306, Alexandria, VA 22314

John Bastyr College of Naturopathic Medicine, 1408 N.E. 45th St., Seattle, WA 98105

National College of Naturopathic Medicine, 11231 S.E. Market St., Portland, OR 97216

Ontario College of Naturopathic Medicine, 60 Berl Avenue, Toronto, Ontario, Canada

Pacific Academy of Homeopathic Medicine, 1678 Shattuck #42, Berkeley, CA 94709

New England School of Homeopathy, 356 Middle St., Amherst, MA 01002

British Institute of Homeopathy, 520 Washington Blvd., #423, Marina del Rey, CA 90292

National Homeopathic Dental Seminars, P.O. Box 123, Marengo, IL 60152

Homeopathic Veterinary Courses, c/o Richard Pitcairn, D.V.M., Ph.D., 1283 Lincoln St., Eugene, OR 97404

For updated listings of addresses and phone numbers of schools and training programs, contact Homeopathic Educational Services, 2124 Kittredge St., Berkeley CA 94704.

ABOUT THE AUTHOR

Dana Ullman, M.P.H., received his Masters in public health from the University of California at Berkeley, specializing in health education. He has been actively educating the general public and the medical community about homeopathic medicine since 1972. He has authored four books, including *Discovering Homeopathy: Medicine for the 21st Century* and *Everybody's Guide to Homeopathic Medicines* (coauthored with Stephen Cummings, M.D.). His company, Homeopathic Educational Services, has published twenty books on homeopathy and is one of America's primary distributors of homeopathic books, tapes, medicines, and software. He is the founder and president of the Foundation for Homeopathic Education and Research in Berkeley, California, and is an elected member of the board of directors of the National Center for Homeopathy in Alexandria, Virginia.

Dana serves on the Board of Advisors of several magazines, including *Natural Health* and *Let's Live,* and is the health book reviewer for the *Utne Reader.*

Most recently, Dana has formulated and serves as a spokesperson for a line of homeopathic products called Medicine From Nature, which are manufactured by Nature's Way.